PHARMACOLOGY – RESEARCH, SAFETY TESTING AND REGULATION

THE PHARMACOLOGICAL GUIDE TO TRASTUZUMAB

PHARMACOLOGY – RESEARCH, SAFETY TESTING AND REGULATION

Additional books and e-books in this series can be found on Nova's website under the Series tab.

Pharmacology – Research, Safety Testing and Regulation

The Pharmacological Guide to Trastuzumab

Dorota Bartusik-Aebisher

and

David Aebisher

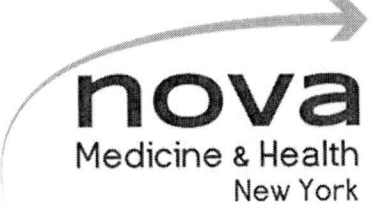

Copyright © 2020 by Nova Science Publishers, Inc.

All rights reserved. No part of this book may be reproduced, stored in a retrieval system or transmitted in any form or by any means: electronic, electrostatic, magnetic, tape, mechanical photocopying, recording or otherwise without the written permission of the Publisher.

We have partnered with Copyright Clearance Center to make it easy for you to obtain permissions to reuse content from this publication. Simply navigate to this publication's page on Nova's website and locate the "Get Permission" button below the title description. This button is linked directly to the title's permission page on copyright.com. Alternatively, you can visit copyright.com and search by title, ISBN, or ISSN.

For further questions about using the service on copyright.com, please contact:
Copyright Clearance Center
Phone: +1-(978) 750-8400 Fax: +1-(978) 750-4470 E-mail: info@copyright.com.

NOTICE TO THE READER

The Publisher has taken reasonable care in the preparation of this book, but makes no expressed or implied warranty of any kind and assumes no responsibility for any errors or omissions. No liability is assumed for incidental or consequential damages in connection with or arising out of information contained in this book. The Publisher shall not be liable for any special, consequential, or exemplary damages resulting, in whole or in part, from the readers' use of, or reliance upon, this material. Any parts of this book based on government reports are so indicated and copyright is claimed for those parts to the extent applicable to compilations of such works.

Independent verification should be sought for any data, advice or recommendations contained in this book. In addition, no responsibility is assumed by the Publisher for any injury and/or damage to persons or property arising from any methods, products, instructions, ideas or otherwise contained in this publication.

This publication is designed to provide accurate and authoritative information with regard to the subject matter covered herein. It is sold with the clear understanding that the Publisher is not engaged in rendering legal or any other professional services. If legal or any other expert assistance is required, the services of a competent person should be sought. FROM A DECLARATION OF PARTICIPANTS JOINTLY ADOPTED BY A COMMITTEE OF THE AMERICAN BAR ASSOCIATION AND A COMMITTEE OF PUBLISHERS.

Additional color graphics may be available in the e-book version of this book.

Library of Congress Cataloging-in-Publication Data

ISBN: 978-1-53617-718-3
Library of Congress Control Number: 2020934571

Published by Nova Science Publishers, Inc. † New York

Contents

Preface		vii
Chapter 1	Trastuzumab: Characteristics	1
Chapter 2	Trastuzumab: Therapeutic Indications	25
Chapter 3	Trastuzumab: Pharmacodynamic Properties	45
Chapter 4	Trastuzumab: Pharmacokinetic Properties	61
Chapter 5	Trastuzumab: Interaction with Other Medicinal Products	101
About the Authors		135
Index		137

PREFACE

This book provides a current review of the field of Trastuzumab pharmacology from a variety of chemical, biochemical, physiological, pharmacokinetical, pharmacodynamical, biophysical and medical perspectives. This book covers breast cancer treatment including current Trastuzumab therapy, radiation therapy and excision of tumors within the limits of healthy tissue. The text presents current knowledge and analysis of pertinent literature and knowledge. This book reports results from experimental models of HER2 oncogene overexpression and treatments which have been used in an effort to understand the relationship between HER2 and response to therapeutics.

In this book the HER2 oncogene has been extensively discussed as a prognostic factor and as a predictor of response to chemotherapy and endocrine therapy. The book includes data regarding the expression of HER2 oncogene in lung cancer and response to trastuzumab alone or in combination with chemotherapeutic agents. The interaction of HER2 with others drugs such as alkylating agents, platinum analogs and topoisomerase inhibitors, as well as additive interactions with taxanes, anthracyclines and some metabolites and antimetabolites are presented. Special cardiological supervision for patients with an increased risk of cardiotoxicity that have hypertension, ischemic heart disease, hypothyroidism or are heavy smokers during adjuvant trastuzumab therapy will also be reviewed.

Chapter 1 - In this chapter, a theoretical overview will be presented concerning qualitative and quantitative composition of trastuzumab, a humanized IgG1 monoclonal antibody produced by mammalian (Chinese hamster ovary) cell suspension culture. The purification of trastuzumab will also be considered and affinity in ion exchange chromatography as well as specific viral inactivation and removal procedures. The pharmaceutical form of Trastuzumab will be discussed.

Chapter 2 - In this chapter Trastuzumab application will be discussed from its initial clinical approval to today. Trastuzumab is used for the treatment of adult patients with HER2 positive metastatic breast cancer and for the treatment of those patients who have received prior chemotherapy. Trastuzumab is indicated for the treatment of adult patients with HER2 positive breast cancer.

Chapter 3 - Trastuzumab is a recombinant humanized IgG1 monoclonal antibody. Overexpression of HER2 is observed in 20%-30% of primary breast cancers, gastric cancer (GC) using immunohistochemistry (IHC) and fluorescence in situ hybridization (FISH) or chromogenic in situ hybridization (CISH) have shown that there is a broad variation of HER2-positivity. In this chapter pharmacodynamic properties of Trastuzumab will be discussed.

Chapter 4 - The pharmacokinetics of trastuzumab will be evaluated in a population pharmacokinetic model analysis using pooled data from patients with HER2 positive tumor types, and healthy volunteers. The case reports and clinical research papers will be discussed.

Chapter 5 - Clinically significant interactions between trastuzumab and concomitant medicinal products used in clinical trials will be discussed. The effects of trastuzumab on the pharmacokinetics of other antineoplastic agents will be reviewed.

Chapter 1

TRASTUZUMAB: CHARACTERISTICS

ABSTRACT

In this chapter, a theoretical overview will be presented concerning qualitative and quantitative composition of trastuzumab, a humanized IgG1 monoclonal antibody produced by mammalian (Chinese hamster ovary) cell suspension culture. The purification of trastuzumab will also be considered and affinity in ion exchange chromatography as well as specific viral inactivation and removal procedures. The pharmaceutical form of Trastuzumab will be discussed.

Keywords: trastuzumab, quantity, quality, purification

HER2 receptor overexpression is found in 20-30% of human breast cancer cases. HER2 is a member of the c-erbB family of receptor tyrosine kinases. HER2 receptor affects the course, treatment and prognosis of breast cancer. Overexpression of the HER2 receptor significantly affects the aggressiveness of cancer. HER2 is an independent adverse prognostic factor and may also predict response to both chemotherapy and endocrine agents (Nevala-Plagemann et al., 2019; Chia et al., 2019; Sethunath et al., 2019; Tahir et al., 2019). Current immunotherapies used in treatment are most often based on monoclonal antibodies such as the Trastuzumab IgG1 class, which has therapeutic effect against the HER2 receptor positive domain. Currently, the biological drug Trastuzumab is considered to be effective only in patients whose cancer is overexpressing HER2. Unfortunately, the exact mechanism of action of Trastuzumab is unknown (Zhao et al., 2019; Walker et al., 2019; Goel et al., 2019; Niikura et al., 2018). This humanized antibody against the extracellular domain of the HER2 receptor binds to the membrane-associated IV subdomain of the extracellular portion of the HER2 protein. By attaching to the receptor, it blocks the cell's ability to transmit signals to the nucleus, thereby slowing the growth of cancer. Cancer cells with HER2 overexpression reproduce at a higher rate due to the higher growth factor (Kataoka et al., 2017; Vollmar et al., 2017; Maruthachalam et al., 2017; Deeks et al., 2017; Chen et al., 2017). The main indications for the implementation of treatment with Trastuzumab are the treatment of HER2 overexpressing breast cancer, palliative treatment, early stage cancer, metastatic breast cancer, and metastatic gastric cancer. In HER2-overexpressing preclinical models, trastuzumab has been shown to have a marked anti-proliferative effect and demonstrates synergy with a number of cytotoxic drugs. Several phase II and phase III clinical trials have now been performed in patients with advanced breast cancer that overexpress HER2 (Wang et al., 2016; Wei et al., 2017; Ilson et al., 2017; Li et al., 2017; Ulaner et al., 2017; Timmer et al., 2017; Soni et al., 2017).

The benefit of Trastuzumab is generally confined to patients whose tumors have gene amplification as detected by fluorescence *in situ* hybridisation (FISH) and this is tightly associated with immunohistochemical (IHC) staining. Trastuzumab has also been shown to be effective when used as first-line monotherapy for advanced breast cancer (Harries et al., 2002; Gabriel et al., 2002). During the past 10 years, significant progress in cancer treatment has been made through the discovery of potent specific and well-tolerated inhibitors of signal transduction. Improved understanding of molecules involved in signal transduction pathways will undoubtedly result in an increasing number of compounds under clinical investigation. Some of the described molecular therapeutic approaches are suitable to enrich the conventional chemotherapy (Gabriel et al., 2002). Statistically significantly higher proportions of patients treated with a combination of trastuzumab and chemotherapy are reported then patients treated by chemotherapy alone (Osoba et al., 2002). Interestingly, overexpression of HER2 does not block binding of other unrelated antibodies of the same isotype (Price-Schiavi et al., 2002). Despite more than four decades of effort, the improvement in survival in metastatic breast cancer has been modest. Recently, however, new drugs such as the taxanes have emerged as pivotal agents in the treatment of metastatic disease and they are now being investigated in the adjuvant setting (Nabholtz et al., 2002; Grillo-López, 2002).

Preliminary results have shown that incorporation of docetaxel can improve the rate of breast preservation surgery and the overall clinical and pathologic complete response rates (Valero et al., 2002). Docetaxel (Taxotere) has been intensively investigated for the treatment of metastatic breast cancer, where it has proved to be one of the most active agents. The consistent demonstration of a high level of efficacy with manageable toxicity ensures the continued widespread investigation of docetaxel in metastatic breast cancer (Esteva, 2002; Wu, 2002). Overexpression of HER2 is common in some nonendocrine tumors, frequently correlates with increased tumor aggressiveness, and can be used as a basis of treatment with trastuzumab. Little is known of its expression in malignant pancreatic endocrine tumors (Goebel et al., 2002). An increasing body of evidence demonstrates that growth factor networks are highly interactive with estrogen receptor signaling in the control of breast cancer growth. As such, tumor responses to antihormones are likely to be a composite of the estrogen receptor and growth factor inhibitory activity of these agents (Nicholson et al., 2002). However, none of these combinations has yet reached the level of an evidence-based standard treatment (Heinemann et al., 2002). This result exemplifies the requirement of employing appropriate matched pair isotopes for imaging and therapy to insure that dosimetry considerations may be addressed accurately (Garmestani et al., 2002; Dicato, 2002). Heregulin-beta1 a combinatorial ligand for human epidermal growth factor receptor 3 (HER3) and HER4, is a regulatory polypeptide having distinct biological effects, such as growth stimulation, differentiation, invasiveness, and migration in mammary epithelial cells

(Talukder et al., 2002). In some studies, notably those in patients with advanced melanoma, significant clinical responses have been observed. Cell-based strategies including autologous tumour cell vaccines, allogeneic tumour cell vaccines and dendritic cell vaccines have been used, and significant responses have been reported in several studies. Few of these methods have so far been applied to breast cancer, but the possible benefits and drawbacks of such an approach will be discussed (Plunkett et al., 2002). However, cardiomyopathies develop in a proportion of patients treated with Trastuzumab, and the incidence of such complications is increased by combination with standard chemotherapy (Ozcelik et al., 2002). These include the receptor tyrosine kinases HER2, the epidermal growth factor receptor. In addition, drugs designed to impede cancer cell invasion and the angiogenic process are also being investigated (Wolff et al., 2002). Current literature suggests two roles for c-erbB-2, either as a pure prognostic factor with no association with therapy or as a factor predictive of benefit from specific types of systemic treatments (Hayes et al., 2002). The overexpression of HER2, a transmembrane glycoprotein tyrosine kinase, has been implicated in mitogenesis, cell survival, invasion and angiogenesis. Two primary mechanisms proposed for the activity of Trastuzumab are downregulation of HER2 and induction of antibody-dependent cell-mediated cytotoxicity (Spiridon et al., 2002; Zinner et al., 2002). The implementation of new drug treatments has improved the prognosis for advanced cancers of the cervix, uterus, and ovary (Daud et al., 2001). Molecularly targeted therapy such as the use of STI571 is one of the first that applies a drug specifically designed to inhibit the product of a constitutively-activating mutation that drives pathogenesis of a solid tumor. Its use can serve as a paradigm for designing molecularly targeted therapies for other malignancies (Blanke et al., 2001). Elucidation of HER2 and its role in malignant transformation has helped define a subset of aggressive breast cancer that may be relatively resistant to non-anthracycline-based therapies and hormonal agents, but responds to targeted molecular therapy. Trastuzumab, an antibody against HER2, has proven effective as single agent therapy in women with HER2 overexpressed metastatic breast cancer. The optimal combination, duration, and sequence of Trastuzumab therapy remain unknown in patients with HER2-positive metastatic disease. The role of continuing treatment after disease progression is also unclear. HER2 status should not be used routinely for clinical decision making regarding hormonal therapy options. Several ongoing trials are attempting to address these and other issues related to HER2 testing to select the most appropriate candidates for these emerging therapies (Spigel et al., 2002). Highly active and well-tolerated therapies, especially those that are justified based on preclinical and neoadjuvant models, represent our best hope for successors to current adjuvant regimens. Such trials are now either in the planning stages or already under way (Tripathy et al., 2002). The combination of gemcitabine and cisplatin has proven effective as first-line chemotherapy for patients with breast cancer, inducing a response rate of 80% in one phase II study (Heinemann et al., 2002). Thus, gemcitabine/trastuzumab resulted in an encouraging 32% response rate, given the heavily pretreated patient population (O'Shaughnessy et al., 2002). Data regarding HER2 expression in lung cancer are more limited, and there is little information regarding HER2 expression and response to trastuzumab alone or in combination with chemotherapeutic agents. Gemcitabine is an active agent against non-small-cell lung cancer and has demonstrated activity in breast cancer as well. *In vitro* modified tetrazolium salt growth assays were performed to determine whether the combination of trastuzumab/gemcitabine produced synergistic or additive effects on breast and lung cancer cell lines. These preclinical studies indicate a need to study the clinical synergistic effects of the gemcitabine/trastuzumab combination in breast cancer patients whose tumors overexpress HER2 (Hirsch et al., 2002). In breast cancer the membrane expression of HER2 receptor protein encoded by the HER2 proto-oncogene seems to have an ever growing clinical significance. In tissue cultures and animal experiments it was shown that the HER2 gene amplification induces malignant transformation and intensifies the aggressiveness of the tumour cells (Tóth et al., 2000; Bánkfalvi et al., 2002). The efficacy of trastuzumab for metastases coupled with the relatively poor prognosis of patients with node-positive, HER2-positive breast cancer has led to the evaluation of trastuzumab as an adjuvant therapy (Roche et al., 2002). Trastuzumab (Herceptin) provides clinical benefits for patients diagnosed with advanced breast cancers that have overexpressed the HER2 protein or have amplified the HER2 gene. This report provides a snapshot of the quality of HER2 assays performed in laboratories nationwide (Paik et al., 2002; Zujewski et al., 2002). The oncogenenic transmembrane tyrosine kinase receptor HER2 is a promising target for treatment of HER2-overexpressing cancers. The humanized anti-HER2 antibody Trastuzumab is under clinical evaluation in combination with chemotherapy against breast cancer (Naruse et al., 2002). Several anticancer drugs have been associated with cardiac toxicity, especially the anthracyclines and trastuzumab. Clinical trials are currently evaluating the role of these markers in predicting both early and late, clinical and subclinical damage associated with anthracyclines and trastuzumab (Sledge et al., 2001). In addition, we have tested the sensitivity of USPC cells to Herceptin treatment. Ten consecutive USPC specimens were assessed by immunohistochemistry for the intensity of expression of HER2. Physiological concentrations of human serum IgG did not inhibit Herceptin-mediated ADCC against USPC. On the basis of these findings and previous reports showing a positive *in vivo* correlation between efficacy of Trastuzumab therapy is an attractive therapeutic strategy in patients harboring chemotherapy-resistant (Isola et al., 2000; Fleck et al., 2002; Bighin et al., 2002; Cimoli et al., 2001; Smith et al., 2001; Piccart-Gebhart et al., 2001; Thomssen et al., 2001). Trastuzumab extends survival in HER2 positive metastatic breast cancer patients when administered with paclitaxel or anthracycline/cyclophosphamide, and the combination with 3-weekly paclitaxel is the current standard first-line therapy. However, other combinations may be equally effective. Weekly paclitaxel plus Trastuzumab has produced responses in 83% of HER2-positive patients treated. Co-administering Trastuzumab with other cytotoxic agents has also been investigated, with combination partners being chosen based on *in vitro* synergy with Trastuzumab, known efficacy as monotherapy and convenience of weekly administration (e.g., docetaxel, vinorelbine). High response rates have been observed in these clinical trials, e.g., up to 80% in combination with vinorelbine. Furthermore, Trastuzumab in combination with weekly paclitaxel, docetaxel or vinorelbine was well tolerated: there was no significant cardiotoxicity or unexpected toxicity and the combination showed an adverse event profile similar to that seen with monotherapy with the cytotoxic agent. Thus, Trastuzumab produces additional clinical benefit when added to all the cytotoxic agents with which it has been examined, further demonstrating its potential for use in HER2-positive breast cancer patients (Leyland-Jones et al., 2001; Crone et al., 2002). In a large-scale clinical trial, treatment with Trastuzumab, a humanized blocking antibody against HER2, led to marked improvement in survival. However, cardiomyopathy was uncovered as a mitigating side effect, thereby suggesting an important role for HER2, signaling as a modifier of human heart failure. To investigate the physiological role of HER2, signaling in the adult heart, we generated mice with a ventricular-restricted deletion of Erbb2. These HER2-deficient conditional mutant mice were viable and displayed no overt phenotype. However, physiological analysis revealed the onset of multiple independent parameters of dilated cardiomyopathy, including chamber dilation, wall thinning and decreased contractility. Additionally, cardiomyocytes isolated from these conditional mutants were more susceptible to anthracycline toxicity (Friedrich, 2002; Tokuda et al., 2002). The HER 2 protein is thought to be a unique and useful molecular target for antibody therapy of cancers overexpressing the HER 2. Some breast cancer patients have responded to trastuzumab alone. Although trastuzumab should not be concurrently used with an anthracycline, cardiotoxicity was also identified in patients treated with trastuzumab alone (Achiwa et al., 2002). Antibodies have for many decades been viewed as ideal molecules for cancer therapy. Although promising from the start, it has taken much of more than two decades to reach the level of clinical application. Many molecular biological and immunological studies have revealed the targeting properties of the host immune system and the biological mechanism of cancer cells for a more specific anticancer effect. Many clinical trials of monoclonal antibodies as a single agent, or in combination protocol with current standard chemotherapy or immunoconjugates have shown promise in the treatment of specific diseases. Furthermore, novel antibody designs and improved understanding of the mode of action of current antibodies lend great hope to the future of this therapeutic approach. The accumulating results from many basic, clinical and translational studies may lead to more individualized therapeutic strategies using these agent directed at specific genetic and immunologic targets (Boér, 2002). The best results are achieved with second-, third-line chemotherapy drugs: capecitabine, vinorelbine, gemcitabine, 5-fluorouracil and a variety of its oral pro-drugs. The combination of chemotherapy with various response modifiers is a rapidly developing field of clinical cancer research. Several other new agents including growth factor receptor antagonists, tumor vaccines, antiangiogenic agents are tested in clinical trials alone and in combination with chemotherapy (Levine, 2000). Epirubicin, a member of the anthracycline family of chemotherapeutic agents, has been widely used throughout the world both as adjuvant therapy in early breast cancer and in metastatic breast cancer. Clinical trials with epirubicin have examined the importance of a dose-response relationship, therapeutic dose, and optimum duration of chemotherapy. Combinations with other chemotherapeutic agents (e.g., epirubicin plus a taxane, sequential or combined use of these agents) are being evaluated in ongoing clinical trials (Mouridsen, 2000). The taxanes paclitaxel and docetaxel have an important role in the treatment of breast cancer, and numerous randomized trials have evaluated their efficacy for this indication. Although a survival benefit was found for taxanes as a component of first-line therapy in two of six trials, the interpretation of both positive trials was confounded by a lack of crossover to taxane therapy in those who were initially randomized to receive standard therapy. The taxanes improve survival in patients with early-stage breast cancer and selected patients with metastatic breast cancer. Further research is necessary in order to identify the efficacy of docetaxel relative to paclitaxel, the optimal dose of docetaxel, the role of weekly taxane therapy, the role of trastuzumab plus taxanes in early-stage disease, and whether taxanes are more effective when given concomitantly or sequentially in patients with early-stage disease (Mamounas, 2000). In patients with operable breast cancer, adjuvant hormonal therapy and adjuvant chemotherapy result in significant and long-term reductions in the rates of disease recurrence and death. These reductions are evident in both patients with node-negative as well as in those with node-positive disease. Neoadjuvant therapy offers the possibility of testing *in vivo* the sensitivity of individual tumors to particular cytotoxic regimens and, hence, of improving ultimate disease control, as well as reducing the extent of local therapy. The contribution and optimal integration of taxanes in the adjuvant setting are yet to be established but are the subject of intense research effort. Similarly, novel targeted therapies such as trastuzumab and bisphosphonates are currently being evaluated in adjuvant studies (Pegram et al., 2001; Tanner et al., 2004; Sato et al., 2005; Koduru et al., 2019; Li et al., 2019; Kaito et al., 2019). Trastuzumab in combination with docetaxel is synergistic *in vitro* (Sauer et al., 2002; Coronella-Wood et al., 2003; Swiatoniowski et al., 2003; Yang et al., 2003; Biganzoli et al., 2004). The development of new chemotherapeutic agents and concepts of radiation therapy, administered as primary, adjuvant and palliative therapy, has led to new perspectives in breast cancer therapy. Apart from conventional chemotherapy, recently developed novel agents interfere with molecular mechanisms that are altered in cancer cells. Promising strategies include inhibition of growth factor receptors, blocking of tumor angiogenesis and signal transduction pathways, modulation of apoptosis, cancer vaccination, and inhibition of invasion and metastasis (Nahta et al., 2002; Zum Büschenfelde et al., 2002; Menendez et al., 2005; Wang et al., 2005; Ramanathan et al., 2005; Chen et al., 2005; Duffy et al., 2005). The monoclonal antibody Trastuzumab (Herceptin) directed against the human epidermal growth factor receptor 2 (HER2) results in tumor regressions when administered to patients with HER2-overexpressing breast cancer. The potentially synergistic activity of HER2-specific antibody and CTL encourages the development of an HER2-targeted immunotherapy using a combination of inhibitory antibodies and CTLs for patients with HER2-overexpressing tumors (Meric et al., 2002; Takehana et al., 2002; (Kaklamani et al., 2004; Beuzeboc, 2004; Harris, 2004; Smith-Jones et al., 2004; Burris et al., 2004; Yaziji et al., 2004; Guarneri et al., 2004; Sundar et al., 2004; Denoux et al., 2003; Risio et al., 2005). The mechanisms of overexpression in gastric adenocarcinomas seem similar to those well-established in breast cancers. Patients having gastric adenocarcinoma with HER2 amplification are potential candidates for a new adjuvant therapy using humanized monoclonal antibody (Park et al., 2002; Campone et al., 2002). Clinical studies showed that paclitaxel is active as single agent and in combination chemotherapy for the management of metastatic breast cancer. A variety of doses and administration schedules have been evaluated in phase II and III trials (Fujimoto-Ouchi et al., 2002). The anti-HER-2 antibody, trastuzumab and the oral fluoropyrimidine, capecitabine (Xeloda), are both effective in breast cancer with different modes of action and toxicity profiles. Therefore, the efficacy in combination therapy of these agents for the treatment of HER-2-overexpressing breast cancer was of interest. An antagonistic interaction *in vitro* between trastuzumab and 5-fluorouracil (5-FUra) in combination has previously been reported. In the same study, the *in vivo* antitumor activity of this combination was investigated (Sawyer et al., 2002). There is an increased incidence of heart failure in patients treated concurrently with anthracyclines and the chemotherapeutic anti-erbB2 agent trastuzumab (de Bono et al., 2002; Morris et al., 2002). The clinical effects of targeting HER in prostate carcinoma are not known. This study explored the feasibility of molecular profiling to determine the correlation between HER-2 expression, hormonal sensitivity, and the antitumor effects of Trastuzumab and paclitaxel in patients with prostate carcinoma. Trastuzumab is not effective as a single agent for the treatment of patients with AI HER2 negative tumors. HER-2 expression varies by clinical state in patients with prostate carcinoma: Accurate HER2 profiling requires sampling metastatic tissue in patients with metastatic disease. Further development of Trastuzumab for the treatment of patients with metastatic prostate carcinoma is not feasible until more reliable and practical methods of sampling metastatic disease are developed to identify patients with HER-2 positive tumors (Esteva et al., 2002). Weekly docetaxel and trastuzumab is an active combination for treating patients with HER2-overexpressing metastatic breast cancer (Wakeling et al., 2001; Fischer et al., 2003; Saeki et al., 2003; Zhang et al., 2000; Tagliabue et al., 2003; Spigel et al., 2003). Furthermore, treatment of wild-type MCF-7 cells with tamoxifen and ZD1839 prevents development of tamoxifen resistance (Izumi et al., 2002). Malignant tumours secrete factors that enable them to commandeer their own blood supply (angiogenesis), and blocking the action of these factors can inhibit tumour growth. But because tumours may become resistant to treatments that target individual angiogenic factors by switching over to other angiogenic molecules, a cocktail of multiple anti-angiogenic agents should be more effective. Here we show that Trastuzumab, a monoclonal antibody against the cell-surface receptor HER2 induces normalization and regression of the vasculature in an experimental human breast tumour that overexpresses HER2 in mice, and that it works by modulating the effects of different pro- and anti-angiogenic factors (Carter et al., 2001; Ullrich et al., 2000; Watanabe et al., 2002). Trastuzumab has provided the first proof that tyrosine kinase modulation, through monoclonal antibodies can translate into improved clinical outcomes in cancer therapy. The development of Trastuzumab was encouraged by the biologic significance of HER2 overexpression. Although the number of patients affected by the targeted molecular abnormality (30% of breast cancer patients) is small and the response rate observed in patients after treated with single agent Trastuzumab is rather low, the ability to document overexpression of the target in breast biopsies, and a growing interest in biologic therapy facilitated the rapid accrual of patients to clinical trials. The challenges of applying research techniques of molecular biology to routine clinical testing have been demonstrated by the experiences with the HER2 oncogene. Immunohistochemistry and fluorescence *in situ* hybridization yielded discrepant results regarding the frequency and degree of HER2 alterations even within the same sample. In order to make the complexity of interpretation of the discrepancy simple, it is wise to build an algorithm to help clinicians follow the ideal sequence of laboratory testings. The experience gained in the testing of Trastuzumab has provided important lessons for the future testing of molecularly targeted compounds (Tokuda, 2003; (Ogura et al., 2003; Cersosimo, 2003; Kim, 2003; Mitchell, 2003; Borchardt et al., 2003).

ACKNOWLEGMENTS

Dorota Bartusik-Aebisher acknowledges support from the National Center of Science NCN (New drug delivery systems-MRI study, Grant OPUS-13 number 2017/25/B/ST4/02481).

REFERENCES

Achiwa, H; Sato, S; Ueda, R. Monoclonal antibody for cancer treatment. *Gan To Kagaku Ryoho.*, 2002, 29(4), 495-501.

Bánkfalvi, A. HER-2 diagnostics. *Magy Onkol.*, 2002, 46(1), 11-5.

Beuzeboc, P. [Indications for Herceptin in breast cancer treatment]. *Gynecol Obstet Fertil.*, 2004 Feb, 32(2), 164-72.

Biganzoli, L; Minisini, A; Aapro, M; Di Leo, A. Chemotherapy for metastatic breast cancer. *Curr Opin Obstet Gynecol.*, 2004, 16(1), 37-41.

Bighin, C; Stevani, I; Venturini, M. Herceptin in elderly patients. *Tumori.*, 2002, 88(1 Suppl 1), S37-8.

Blanke, CD; Eisenberg, BL; Heinrich, MC. Gastrointestinal stromal tumors. *Curr Treat Options Oncol.*, 2001, 2(6), 485-91.

Boér, K. Current trends in pharmacotherapy of breast cancer. *Orv Hetil.*, 2002, 143(14), 725-30. Review. Hungarian.

Borchardt, PE; Yuan, RR; Miederer, M; McDevitt, MR; Scheinberg, DA. Targeted actinium-225 *in vivo* generators for therapy of ovarian cancer. *Cancer Res.*, 2003, Aug 15, 63(16), 5084-90.

Burris, H; 3rd, Yardley, D; Jones, S; Houston, G; Broome, C; Thompson, D; Greco, FA; White, M; Hainsworth, J. Phase II trial of trastuzumab followed by weekly paclitaxel/carboplatin as first-line treatment for patients with metastatic breast cancer. *J Clin Oncol.*, 2004, 22(9), 1621-9.

Campone, M; Fumoleau, P. [Weekly administration of paclitaxel in the treatment of metastatic breast cancer: from rational to practice]. Bull Cancer., 2002, 89(3), 275-82.

Carter, P. Improving the efficacy of antibody-based cancer therapies. Nat Rev Cancer., 2001, 1(2), 118-29.

Cersosimo, RJ. Monoclonal antibodies in the treatment of cancer, Part 1. Am J Health Syst Pharm., 2003, 60(15), 1531-48. Review.

Chen, EX; Siu, LL. Development of molecular targeted anticancer agents, successes, failures and future directions. Curr Pharm Des., 2005, 11(2), 265-72. Revie

Chen, W; Li, X; Zhu, L; Liu, J; Xu, W; Wang, P. Preclinical and clinical applications of specific molecular imaging for HER2-positive breast cancer. Cancer Biol Med., 2017, 14(3), 271-280.

Cimoli, G; Bagnasco, L; Pescarolo, MP; Avignolo, C; Melchiori, A; Pasa, S; Biasotti, B; Taningher, M; Parodi, S. Signaling proteins as innovative targets for antineoplastic therapy: our experience with the signaling protein c-myc. Tumori., 2001, 87(6), S20-3.

Coronella-Wood, JA; Hersh, EM. Naturally occurring B-cell responses to breast cancer. Cancer Immunol Immunother., 2003, 52(12), 715-38.

Crone, SA; Zhao, YY; Fan, L; Gu, Y; Minamisawa, S; Liu, Y; Peterson, KL; Chen, J; Kahn, R; Condorelli, G; Ross, J; Jr. Chien, KR; Lee, KF. ErbB2 is essential in the prevention of dilated cardiomyopathy. Nat Med., 2002, 8(5), 459-65.

Daud, A; Munster, P; Munster, P; Spriggs, DR. New drugs in gynecologic cancer. Curr Treat Options Oncol., 2001, 2(2), 119-28.

de Bono, JS; Rowinsky, EK. The ErbB receptor family: a therapeutic target for cancer. Trends Mol Med., 2002, 8(4 Suppl), S19-26.

Deeks, ED. Neratinib: First Global Approval. Drugs., 2017, 77(15), 1695-1704.

Denoux, Y; Arnould, L; Fiche, M; Lannes, B; Couturier, J; Vincent-Salomon, A; Penault-Llorca, F; Antoine, M; Balaton, A; Baranzelli, MC; Becette, V; Bellocq, JP; Bibeau, F; Ettore, F; Fridman, V; Gnassia, JP; Jacquemier, J; MacGrogan, G; Mathieu, MC; Migeon, C; Rigaud, C; Roger, P; Sigal-Zafrani, B; Simony-Lafontaine, J; Trassard,

M; Treilleux, I; Verriele, V; Voigt, JJ. Groupe d'Etude des Facteurs Pronostiques en Immunohistochimie dans le Cancer du Sein. [HER2 gene amplification assay: is CISH an alternative to FISH?]. *Ann Pathol.*, 2003, 23(6), 617-22.

Dicato, M. High-dose chemotherapy in breast cancer: where are we now? *Semin Oncol.*, 2002, 29(3 Suppl 8), 16-20.

Duffy, MJ. Predictive markers in breast and other cancers: a review. *Clin Chem.*, 2005, 51(3), 494-503

Esmaeli, B; Hortobagyi, GN; Esteva, FJ; Booser, D; Ahmadi, MA; Rivera, E; Arbuckle, R; Delpassand, E; Guerra, L; Valero, V. Canalicular stenosis secondary to weekly versus every-3-weeks docetaxel in patients with metastatic breast cancer. *Ophthalmology.*, 2002, Jun, 109(6), 1188-91.

Esteva, FJ; Valero, V; Booser, D; Guerra, LT; Murray, JL; Pusztai, L; Cristofanilli, M; Arun, B; Esmaeli, B; Fritsche, HA; Sneige, N; Smith, TL; Hortobagyi, GN. Phase II study of weekly docetaxel and trastuzumab for patients with HER-2-overexpressing metastatic breast cancer. *J Clin Oncol.*, 2002, Apr 1, 20(7), 1800-8.

Esteva, FJ. The current status of docetaxel for metastatic breast cancer. *Oncology* (Williston Park)., 2002, 16(6 Suppl 6), 17-26.

Fischer, OM; Streit, S; Hart, S; Ullrich, A. Beyond Herceptin and Gleevec. *Curr Opin Chem Biol.*, 2003,7(4), 490-5.

Fleck, LM. Rationing: don't give up. *Hastings Cent Rep.*, 2002, 32(2), 35-6.

Friedrich, MJ. Cardiotoxicity concerns prompt data review in breast cancer trial. *J Natl Cancer Inst.*, 2002, 94(9), 650-1.

Fujimoto-Ouchi, K; Sekiguchi, F; Tanaka, Y. Antitumor activity of combinations of anti-HER-2 antibody trastuzumab and oral fluoropyrimidines capecitabine/5'-dFUrd in human breast cancer models. *Cancer Chemother Pharmacol.*, 2002, 49(3), 211-6.

Gabriel, B; Fischer, DC; Kieback, DG. Molecular mechanisms in signal transduction: new targets for the therapy of gynecologic malignancies. *Onkologie.*, 2002, 25(3), 240-7.

Garmestani, K; Milenic, DE; Plascjak, PS; Brechbiel, MW. A new and convenient method for purification of 86Y using a Sr(II) selective resin and comparison of biodistribution of 86Y and 111In labeled Herceptin. *Nucl Med Biol.*, 2002, 29(5), 599-606.

Goebel, SU; Iwamoto, M; Raffeld, M; Gibril, F; Hou, W; Serrano, J; Jensen, RT. Her-2/neu expression and gene amplification in gastrinomas: correlations with tumor biology, growth, and aggressiveness. *Cancer Res.*, 2002, 62(13), 3702-10.

Grillo-López, AJ. AntiCD20 mAbs: modifying therapeutic strategies and outcomes in the treatment of lymphoma patients. *Expert Rev Anticancer Ther.*, 2002, 2(3), 323-9.

Guarneri, V; Conte, PF. The curability of breast cancer and the treatment of advanced disease. *Eur J Nucl Med Mol Imaging.*, 2004 Jun, 31 Suppl 1, S149-61. Epub 2004 Apr 24.

Harries, M; Smith, I. The development and clinical use of trastuzumab (Herceptin). *Endocr Relat Cancer.*, 2002, 9(2), 75-85.

Harris, M. Monoclonal antibodies as therapeutic agents for cancer. *Lancet Oncol.*, 2004 May, 5(5), 292-302. Review.

Hayes, DF; Thor, AD. c-erbB-2 in breast cancer: development of a clinically useful marker. *Semin Oncol.*, 2002, 29(3), 231-45.

Heinemann, V. Gemcitabine plus cisplatin for the treatment of metastatic breast cancer. *Clin Breast Cancer.*, 2002, Suppl 1, 24-9.

Heinemann, V. Present and future treatment of pancreatic cancer. *Semin Oncol.*, 2002, 29(3 Suppl 9), 23-31.

Hirsch, FR; Franklin, WA; Bunn, PA. What is the role of HER-2/neu and trastuzumab (Herceptin) in lung cancer? *Lung Cancer.*, 2002, 36(3), 263-4.

Hirsch, FR; Helfrich, B; Franklin, WA; Varella-Garcia, M; Chan, DC; Bunn, PA. Jr. Preclinical studies of gemcitabine and trastuzumab in breast and lung cancer cell lines. *Clin Breast Cancer.*, 2002, 3 Suppl, 1, 12-6.

Ilson, DH. Advances in the treatment of gastric cancer. *Curr Opin Gastroenterol.*, 2017, 33(6), 473-476.

Isola, J; Järvinen, T; Tanner, M; Holli, K. HER-2/neu oncogene in the selection of treatment for breast cancer and as a target of immunotherapy. *Duodecim.*, 2000, 116(15), 1538-46.

Izumi, Y; Xu, L; di Tomaso, E; Fukumura, D; Jain, RK. Tumour biology: herceptin acts as an anti-angiogenic cocktail. *Nature.*, 2002, 416(6878), 279-80.

Kaito, A; Kuwata, T; Tokunaga, M; Shitara, K; Sato, R; Akimoto, T; Kinoshita, T. HER2 heterogeneity is a poor prognosticator for HER2-positive gastric cancer. *World J Clin Cases.*, 2019, 7(15), 1964-1977.

Kaklamani, V; O'Regan, RM. New targeted therapies in breast cancer. *Semin Oncol.*, 2004, 31(2 Suppl 4), 20-5.

Kataoka, K; Deleersnijder, A; Lordick, F. Will molecular target agents enable the multidisciplinary treatment in stage IV gastric cancer? *Eur J Surg Oncol.*, 2017, 43(10), 1835-1845.

Kikuchi, T; Shimizu, H; Akiyama, Y; Taniguchi, S. In situ delivery and production system of trastuzumab scFv with Bifidobacterium. *Biochem Biophys Res Commun.*, 2017, 493(1), 306-312.

Kim, JA. Targeted therapies for the treatment of cancer. *Am J Surg.*, 2003, 186(3), 264-8.

Koduru, P; Chen, W; Haley, B; Ho, K; Oliver, D; Wilson, K. Cytogenomic characterization of double minute heterogeneity in therapy related acute myeloid leukemia. *Cancer Genet.*, 2019, 238, 69-75.

Levine, M. Epirubicin in breast cancer: present and future. *Clin Breast Cancer.*, 2000, 1 Suppl 1, S62-7.

Leyland-Jones, B. Maximizing the response to Herceptin therapy through optimal use and patient selection. *Anticancer Drugs.*, 2001, 12 Suppl, 4, S11-7.

Li, Y; Family, L; Yang, SJ; Klippel, Z; Page, JH; Chao, C. Risk of Febrile Neutropenia Associated With Select Myelosuppressive Chemotherapy Regimens in a Large Community-Based Oncology Practice. *J Natl Compr Canc Netw.*, 2017, 15(9), 1122-1130.

Mamounas, EP. Present state and future prospects: a review of cooperative groups' adjuvant and neoadjuvant trials in breast cancer. *Clin Breast Cancer.*, 2001, 2 Suppl 1, S20-30.

Mandler, R; Kobayashi, H; Davis, MY; Waldmann, TA; Brechbiel, MW. Modifications in synthesis strategy improve the yield and efficacy of geldanamycin-herceptin immunoconjugates. *Bioconjug Chem.*, 2002, 13(4), 786-91.

Maruthachalam, BV; El-Sayed, A; Liu, J; Sutherland, AR; Hill, W; Alam, MK; Pastushok, L; Fonge, H; Barreto, K; Geyer, CR. A Single-Framework Synthetic Antibody Library Containing a Combination of Canonical and Variable Complementarity-Determining Regions. *Chembiochem.*, 2017, 18(22), 2247-2259.

Menendez, JA; Vellon, L; Colomer, R; Lupu, R. Oleic acid, the main monounsaturated fatty acid of olive oil, suppresses Her-2/neu (erbB-2) expression and synergistically enhances the growth inhibitory effects of trastuzumab (Herceptin) in breast cancer cells with Her-2/neu oncogene amplification. *Ann Oncol.*, 2005, 16(3), 359-71.

Meric, F; Hung, MC; Hortobagyi, GN; Hunt, KK. HER2/neu in the management of invasive breast cancer. *J Am Coll Surg.*, 2002, 194(4), 488-501.

Mitchell, MS. Combinations of anticancer drugs and immunotherapy. *Cancer Immunol Immunother.*, 2003, 52(11), 686-92.

Mitsumori, M. Current status of radiation therapy--evidence-based medicine (EBM) of radiation therapy. Breast cancer. *Nihon Igaku Hoshasen Gakkai Zasshi.*, 2002, 62(4), 138-43.

Morris, MJ; Reuter, VE; Kelly, WK; Slovin, SF; Kenneson, K; Verbel, D; Osman, I; Scher, HI. HER-2 profiling and targeting in prostate carcinoma. *Cancer.*, 2002, 94(4), 980-6.

Mouridsen, HT. Rationale and use of epirubicin-based therapy in the adjuvant setting. *Clin Breast Cancer.*, 2000, 1 Suppl, 1, S34-40.

Nabholtz, JM; Reese, DM; Lindsay, MA; Riva, A. Combination chemotherapy for metastatic breast cancer. *Expert Rev Anticancer Ther.*, 2002, 2(2), 169-80.

Nahta, R; Iglehart, JD; Kempkes, B; Schmidt, EV. Rate-limiting effects of Cyclin D1 in transformation by ErbB2 predicts synergy between herceptin and flavopiridol. *Cancer Res.*, 2002, 62(8), 2267-71.

Naruse, I; Fukumoto, H; Saijo, N; Nishio, K. Enhanced anti-tumor effect of trastuzumab in combination with cisplatin. *Jpn J Cancer Res.*, 2002, 93(5), 574-81.

Nevala-Plagemann, C; Moser, J; Gilcrease, GW; Garrido-Laguna, I. Survival of patients with metastatic HER2 positive gastro-oesophageal cancer treated with second-line chemotherapy plus trastuzumab or ramucirumab after progression on front-line chemotherapy plus trastuzumab. *ESMO Open.*, 2019, 4(4), e000539.

Nicholson, RI; Hutcheson, IR; Harper, ME; Knowlden, JM; Barrow, D; McClelland, RA; Jones, HE; Wakeling, AE; Gee, JM. Modulation of epidermal growth factor receptor in endocrine-resistant, estrogen-receptor-positive breast cancer. *Ann N Y Acad Sci.*, 2002 Jun, 963, 104-15.

Niikura, N; Shimomura, A; Fukatsu, Y; Sawaki, M; Ogiya, R; Yasojima, H; Fujisawa T; Yamamoto, M; Tsuneizumi, M; Kitani, A; Watanabe, J; Matsui, A; Takahashi, Y; Takashima, S; Shien, T; Tamura, K; Saji, S; Masuda, N; Tokuda, Y; Iwata, H. Durable complete response in HER2-positive breast cancer: a multicenter retrospective analysis. *Breast Cancer Res Treat.*, 2018, 167(1), 81-87.

Ogura, H; Akiyama, F; Kasumi, F; Kazui, T; Sakamoto, G. Evaluation of HER-2 status in breast carcinoma by fluorescence *in situ* hybridization and immunohistochemistry. *Breast Cancer.*, 2003, 10(3), 234-40.

O'Shaughnessy, J; Vukelja, SJ; Marsland, T; Kimmel, G; Ratnam, S; Pippen, J. Phase II trial of gemcitabine plus trastuzumab in metastatic breast cancer patients previously treated with chemotherapy: preliminary results. *Clin Breast Cancer.*, 2002, 3 Suppl 1, 17-20.

Ozcelik, C; Erdmann, B; Pilz, B; Wettschureck, N; Britsch, S; Hübner, N; Chien, KR; Birchmeier, C; Garratt, AN. Conditional mutation of the ErbB2 (HER2) receptor in cardiomyocytes leads to dilated cardiomyopathy. *Proc Natl Acad Sci U S A.*, 2002, 99(13), 8880-5. Epub 2002 Jun 18.

Paik, S; Bryant, J; Tan-Chiu, E; Romond, E; Hiller, W; Park, K; Brown, A; Yothers, G; Anderson, S; Smith, R; Wickerham, DL; Wolmark, N. Real-world performance of HER2 testing--National Surgical Adjuvant

Breast and Bowel Project experience. *J Natl Cancer Inst.*, 2002, 94(11), 852-4.

Park, JW; Hong, K; Kirpotin, DB; Colbern, G; Shalaby, R; Baselga, J; Shao, Y; Nielsen, UB; Marks, JD; Moore, D; Papahadjopoulos, D; Benz, CC. Anti-HER2 immunoliposomes: enhanced efficacy attributable to targeted delivery. *Clin Cancer Res.*, 2002, 8(4), 1172-81.

Pegram, MD; O'Callaghan, C. Combining the anti-HER2 antibody trastuzumab with taxanes in breast cancer: results and trial considerations. *Clin Breast Cancer.*, 2001, 2 Suppl 1, S15-9.

Piccart-Gebhart, MJ. Herceptin: the future in adjuvant breast cancer therapy. *Anticancer Drugs.*, 2001, 12 Suppl 4, S27-33.

Plunkett, TA; Miles, DW. New biological therapies for breast cancer. *Int J Clin Pract.*, 2002 May, 56(4), 261-6. Review.

Price-Schiavi, SA; Jepson, S; Li, P; Arango, M; Rudland, PS; Yee, L; Carraway, KL. Rat Muc4 (sialomucin complex) reduces binding of anti-ErbB2 antibodies to tumor cell surfaces, a potential mechanism for herceptin resistance. *Int J Cancer.*, 2002, 99(6), 783-91.

Ramanathan, RK; Hwang, JJ; Zamboni, WC; Sinicrope, FA; Safran, H; Wong, MK; Earle, M; Brufsky, A; Evans, T; Troetschel, M; Walko, C; Day, R; Chen, HX; Finkelstein, S. Low overexpression of HER-2/neu in advanced colorectal cancer limits the usefulness of trastuzumab (Herceptin) and irinotecan as therapy. A phase II trial. *Cancer Invest.*, 2004, 22(6), 858-65.

Risio. M; Casorzo. L; Redana. S; Montemurro. F. HER2 gene-amplified breast cancers with monosomy of chromosome 17 are poorly responsive to trastuzumab-based treatment. *Oncol Rep.*, 2005, 13(2), 305-9.

Roche, PC; Suman, VJ; Jenkins, RB; Davidson, NE; Martino, S; Kaufman, PA; Addo, FK; Murphy, B; Ingle, JN; Perez, EA. Concordance between local and central laboratory HER2 testing in the breast intergroup trial N9831. *J Natl Cancer Inst.*, 2002, 94(11), 855-7.

Saeki, T; Takashima, S. [Clinical implications of trastuzumab]. *Gan To Kagaku Ryoho.*, 2003 Aug, 30(8), 1094-9.

Santin, AD; Bellone, S; Gokden, M; Palmieri, M; Dunn, D; Agha, J; Roman, JJ; Hutchins, L; Pecorelli, S; O'Brien, T; Cannon, MJ; Parham, GP. Overexpression of HER-2/neu in uterine serous papillary cancer. *Clin Cancer Res.*, 2002, 8(5), 1271-9.

Sato, S; Kajiyama, Y; Sugano, M; Iwanuma, Y; Sonoue, H; Matsumoto, T; Sasai, K; Tsurumaru, M. Monoclonal antibody to HER-2/neu receptor enhances radiosensitivity of esophageal cancer cell lines expressing HER-2/neu oncoprotein. *Int J Radiat Oncol Biol Phys..* 2005. 61(1), 203-11.

Sauer, G; Deissler, H; Kurzeder, C; Kreienberg, R. New molecular targets of breast cancer therapy. *Strahlenther Onkol.*, 2002, 178(3), 123-33.

Sawyer, DB; Zuppinger, C; Miller, TA; Eppenberger, HM; Suter, TM. Modulation of anthracycline-induced myofibrillar disarray in rat ventricular myocytes by neuregulin-1beta and anti-erbB2: potential mechanism for trastuzumab-induced cardiotoxicity. *Circulation.*, 2002, 105(13), 1551-4.

Sledge, GW. Jr. Breast cancer in the clinic: treatments past, treatments future. *J Mammary Gland Biol Neoplasia.*, 2001, 6(4), 487-95.

Smith, IE. Efficacy and safety of Herceptin in women with metastatic breast cancer: results from pivotal clinical studies. *Anticancer Drugs.*, 2001, 12, Suppl 4, S3-10.

Smith-Jones, PM; Solit, DB. Generation of DOTA-conjugated antibody fragments for radioimmunoimaging. *Methods Enzymol.*, 2004, 386, 262-75.

Soni, KS; Lei, F; Desale, SS; Marky, LA; Cohen, SM; Bronich, TK. Tuning polypeptide-based micellar carrier for efficient combination therapy of ErbB2-positive breast cancer. *J Control Release.*, 2017, 264, 276-287.

Sparano, JA; Brown, DL; Wolff, AC. Predicting cancer therapy-induced cardiotoxicity: the role of troponins and other markers. *Drug Saf.*, 2002, 25(5), 301-11.

Spigel, DR; Burstein, HJ. HER2 overexpressing metastatic breast cancer. *Curr Treat Options Oncol.*, 2002, 3(2), 163-74.

Spigel, DR. HER2 and surgery: more questions to answer. *Lancet.*, 2003, 362(9383), 502-3.

Spiridon, CI; Ghetie, MA; Uhr, J; Marches, R; Li, JL; Shen, GL; Vitetta, ES. Targeting multiple Her-2 epitopes with monoclonal antibodies results in improved antigrowth activity of a human breast cancer cell line *in vitro* and *in vivo*. *Clin Cancer Res.*, 2002, 8(6), 1720-30.

Sundar, S; Decatris, MP; O'Byrne, KJ. Management of endocrine resistant breast cancer. *J Br Menopause Soc.*, 2004, 10(1), 16-23.

Swiatoniowski, G; Dabrowska, M; Kłaniewski, T; Molenda, W. [Erb-2 overexpression in breast cancer. *Ginekol Pol.*, 2003, 74(4), 332-8.

Tagliabue, E; Agresti, R; Carcangiu, ML; Ghirelli, C; Morelli, D; Campiglio, M; Martel, M; Giovanazzi, R; Greco, M; Balsari, A; Ménard, S. Role of HER2 in wound-induced breast carcinoma proliferation. *Lancet.*, 2003, 362(9383), 527-33.

Tahir, H; Bardia, N; Bath, K; Ahmed, Y; Rafique, M; Omar, B; Malozzi, C. Trastuzumab-Induced Cardiomyopathy and Intermittent Left Bundle Branch Block. *Cardiol Res.*, 2019, 10(4), 230-235.

Takehana, T; Kunitomo, K; Kono, K; Kitahara, F; Iizuka, H; Matsumoto, Y; Fujino, MA; Ooi, A. Status of c-erbB-2 in gastric adenocarcinoma: a comparative study of immunohistochemistry, fluorescence *in situ* hybridization and enzyme-linked immuno-sorbent assay. *Int J Cancer.*, 2002, 98(6), 833-7.

Talukder, AH; Wang, RA; Kumar, R. Expression and transactivating functions of the bZIP transcription factor GADD153 in mammary epithelial cells. *Oncogene.*, 2002, 21(27), 4289-300.

Tanner, M; Kapanen, AI; Junttila, T; Raheem, O; Grenman, S; Elo, J; Elenius, K; Isola, J. Characterization of a novel cell line established from a patient with Herceptin-resistant breast cancer. *Mol Cancer Ther.*, 2004, 3(12), 1585-92

Thomssen, C. Trials of new combinations of Herceptin in metastatic breast cancer. *Anticancer Drugs.*, 2001, 12, Suppl 4, S19-25.

Timmer, M; Werner, JM; Röhn, G; Ortmann, M; Blau, T; Cramer, C; Stavrinou, P; Krischek, B; Mallman, P; Goldbrunner, R. Discordance and Conversion Rates of Progesterone-, Estrogen-, and HER2/neu-

Receptor Status in Primary Breast Cancer and Brain Metastasis Mainly Triggered by Hormone Therapy. *Anticancer Res.*, 2017, 37(9), 4859-4865.

Tokuda, Y; Suzuki, Y; Saitou, Y; Ohta, M; Tajima, T. [Trastuzumab (Herceptin)]. *Gan To Kagaku Ryoho.*, 2002, 29(4), 645-52.

Tokuda, Y. Antibodies as molecular target-based therapy: trastuzumab. *Int J Clin Oncol.*, 2003, 8(4), 224-9.

Tóth, J; Szentkuti, A. Expression of HER2 in breast cancer. *Magy Onkol.*, 2000, 44(1), 39-51.

Tripathy, D. Gemcitabine in breast cancer: future directions. *Clin Breast Cancer.*, 2002, Suppl 1, 45-8.

Ulaner, GA; Hyman, DM; Lyashchenko, SK; Lewis, JS; Carrasquillo, JA. 89Zr-Trastuzumab PET/CT for Detection of Human Epidermal Growth Factor Receptor 2-Positive Metastases in Patients With Human Epidermal Growth Factor Receptor 2-Negative Primary Breast Cancer. *Clin Nucl Med.*, 2017, 42(12), 912-917.

Ullrich, A. Axel Ullrich--a pioneer in gene technology. Interviewed by Ezzie Hutchinson. *Lancet Oncol.*, 2000, 1(1), 50-3.

Valero, V. Primary chemotherapy with docetaxel for the management of breast cancer. *Oncology* (Williston Park)., 2002, 16(6 Suppl 6), 35-43.

Vollmar, BS; Wei, B; Ohri, R; Zhou, J; He, J; Yu, SF; Leipold, D; Cosino, E; Yee, S; Fourie-O'Donohue, A; Li, G; Phillips, GL; Kozak, KR; Kamath, A; Xu, K; Lee, G; Lazar, GA; Erickson, HK. Attachment Site Cysteine Thiol pKa Is a Key Driver for Site-Dependent Stability of THIOMAB Antibody-Drug Conjugates. *Bioconjug Chem.*, 2017, 28(10), 2538-2548.

Wakeling, AE; Nicholson, RI; Gee, JM. Prospects for combining hormonal and nonhormonal growth factor inhibition. *Clin Cancer Res.*, 2001, Dec, 7(12 Suppl), 4350s-4355s, discussion 4411s-4412s.

Wang, L; Yu, X; Wang, C; Pan, S; Liang, B; Zhang, Y; Chong, X; Meng, Y; Dong, J; Zhao, Y; Yang, Y; Wang, H; Gao, J; Wei, H; Zhao, J; Wang, H; Hu, C; Xiao, W; Li, B. The anti-ErbB2 antibody H2-18 and the pan-PI3K inhibitor GDC-0941 effectively inhibit trastuzumab-resistant ErbB2-overexpressing breast cancer. *Oncotarget.*, 2016, 8(32), 52877-52888.

Watanabe, T; Katsumata, N; Ando, M; Mukai, H; Shimizu, C; Kitagawa, R; Saijo, NG. [Genetic testing for effective Herceptin therapy]. *Nihon Rinsho.*, 2002, 60(3), 603-11. Review. Japanese.

Wei, H; Cai, H; Jin, Y; Wang, P; Zhang, Q; Lin, Y; Wang, W; Cheng, J; Zeng, N; Xu, T; Zhou, A. Structural basis of a novel heterodimeric Fc for bispecific antibody production. *Oncotarget.*, 2017, 8(31), 51037-51049.

Wolff, RA. Exploiting molecular targets in pancreatic cancer. *Hematol Oncol Clin North Am.*, 2002,16(1), 139-57.

Wu, JT. C-erbB2 oncoprotein and its soluble ectodomain: a new potential tumor marker for prognosis early detection and monitoring patients undergoing Herceptin treatment. *Clin Chim Acta.*, 2002, 322(1-2), 11-9.

Yang, Z; Bagheri-Yarmand, R; Balasenthil, S; Hortobagyi, G; Sahin, AA; Barnes, CJ; Kumar, R. HER2 regulation of peroxisome proliferator-activated receptor gamma (PPARgamma) expression and sensitivity of breast cancer cells to PPARgamma ligand therapy. *Clin Cancer Res.*, 2003, 9(8), 3198-203.

Yaziji, H; Goldstein, LC; Barry, TS; Werling, R; Hwang, H; Ellis, GK; Gralow, JR; Livingston, RB; Gown, AM. HER-2 testing in breast cancer using parallel tissue-based methods. *JAMA.*, 2004, 291(16), 1972-7.

Zhang, HT; Wang, Q; Greene, MI; Murali, R. New perspectives on anti-HER2/neu therapeutics. *Drug News Perspect.*, 2000, 13(6), 325-9.

Zhao, S; Liu, XY; Jin, X; Ma, D; Xiao, Y; Shao, ZM; Jiang, YZ. Molecular portraits and trastuzumab responsiveness of estrogen receptor-positive: progesterone receptor-positive: and HER2-positive breast cancer. *Theranostics.*, 2019, 9(17), 4935-4945.

Zinner, RG; Kim, J; Herbst, RS. Non-small cell lung cancer clinical trials with trastuzumab: their foundation and preliminary results. *Lung Cancer.*, 2002, 37(1), 17-27.

Zujewski, JA. Build quality in"--HER2 testing in the real world. *J Natl Cancer Inst.*, 2002, 94(11), 788-9.

zum Büschenfelde, CM; Hermann, C; Schmidt, B; Peschel, C; Bernhard, H. Antihuman epidermal growth factor receptor 2 (HER2) monoclonal antibody trastuzumab enhances cytolytic activity of class I-restricted HER2-specific T lymphocytes against HER2-overexpressing tumor cells. *Cancer Res.*, 2002, 62(8), 2244-7.

Chapter 2

TRASTUZUMAB: THERAPEUTIC INDICATIONS

ABSTRACT

In this chapter Trastuzumab application will be discussed from its initial clinical approval to today. Trastuzumab is used for the treatment of adult patients with HER2 positive metastatic breast cancer and for the treatment of those patients who have received prior chemotherapy. Trastuzumab is indicated for the treatment of adult patients with HER2 positive breast cancer.

Keywords: trastuzumab, positive metastatic breast cancer, early breast cancer

The HER2 protein is thought to be a target for antibody therapy for cancers overexpressing the HER2/neu gene (Tokuda et al., 2002). Trastuzumab has been shown to inhibit the proliferation of human tumor cells that overexpress HER2 and to be a mediator of antibody-dependent cellular toxicity (Ebi et al., 2002; Rowinsky, 2003; Rivera, 2003; Kubo et al., 2003; Theodoulou et al., 2003; Grossi et al., 2003). There is therefore a need for new, modified anticancer therapies. Trastuzumab is the first clinically available oncogene-targeted therapeutic agent for treatment of solid tumours. First-line trastuzumab in combination with chemotherapy, particularly paclitaxel, significantly improved time to disease progression, duration of response, and time to treatment failure (Leyland-Jones, 2002; Hsu et al., 2002). As combinations and sequences of anthracyclines and taxanes increasingly become standard adjuvant treatment for early breast cancer, a major need for new treatment options for metastatic breast cancer will arise. Vinorelbine is highly active in the treatment of metastatic breast cancer, both as a single agent and in combination regimens. Furthermore, it is well tolerated, with a low incidence of subjective toxicities. It is anticipated, therefore, that vinorelbine will become increasingly utilized for treating metastatic breast cancer due to its favorable safety profile, good tolerability, and promising results in combination with other chemotherapy agents (Domenech et al., 2001; (Ibrahim et al., 2001; Laufman et al., 2001; Goldman, 2003; Lu et al., 2004; Kauraniemi et al., 2004; Nihira, 2003; Aprikian et al., 2003). Combinations with cisplatin have been investigated, essentially, as salvage therapy for patients. The combinations of cisplatin with older pharmacological agents (5-fluorouracil, etoposide) have moderate activity, while the combinations of cisplatin with the newer agents (vinorelbine, paclitaxel, docetaxel, gemcitabine) appear to be more active (Martín, 2001; Urruticoechea et al., 2017; Kitayama et al., 2017; van Ramshorst et al., 2017; Zer et al., 2017). The taxanes paclitaxel and docetaxel have an important role in the treatment of breast cancer. The taxanes improve survival in patients with early-stage breast cancer and selected patients with metastatic breast cancer. Further research is necessary in order to identify the efficacy of docetaxel relative to paclitaxel, the optimal dose of docetaxel, the role of weekly taxane therapy, the role of trastuzumab plus taxanes in early-stage disease, and whether taxanes are more effective when given concomitantly or sequentially in patients with early-stage disease (Sparano, 2000; Robins et al., 2002; De Iuliis et al., 2017; Curigliano et al., 2017; Tran et al., 2017; Kim et al., 2017). The management of metastatic breast cancer is changing as a consequence of extraordinary discoveries in cancer research and the development of more advanced diagnostic technologies. Although traditional chemotherapeutics such as anthracyclines and taxanes still represent the mainstay of treatment for this disease, new drugs are demonstrating significant clinical activity and sometimes a better toxicity profile (Cristofanilli et al., 2001). Preclinical data suggests a role for trastuzumab in the treatment of non-small cell lung cancer. HER2 protein is overexpressed in 20% to 66% of resected NSCLC tumors, and has been shown to predict poor patient outcome in multiple series (Rivera, 2003; Kubo et al., 2003; Theodoulou et al., 2003). Despite intensive treatment efforts, the prognosis for lung cancer is very poor; less than 15% of patients survive 5 years. Prospective clinical studies with trastuzumab in lung cancer are ongoing. Future studies in NSCLC need to include immunohistochemistry and fluorescence in situ hybridization analysis to determine the method of choice for evaluating clinically relevant HER2/neu-positive tumors (Hirsch et al., 2002). Gemcitabine was identified as an active agent in the treatment of urothelial cancer early in its clinical development. Combinations with targeted therapeutic agents such as the epidermal growth factor receptor inhibitors and trastuzumab have great potential, but the clinical studies have not yet been completed (Stadler et al., 2002). The main focus of the present study was to assess the efficacy of interphase cytogenetics using fluorescence in situ hybridization as a valid alternative to immunohistochemistry in paraffin-embedded tissue sections and/or the efficacy of the combination of the two methods, while, at the same time, aiming to provide additional information on the use of the two methods (Cianciulli et al., 2002; Azzoli et al., 2002 (Sledge, 2003; Gori et al., 2004; Ganne et al., 2003; Bouchie, 2004; Cobleigh et al., 2004; Lu et al., 2004; van Zanten et al., 2004; Ross et al., 2003; Sun et al., 2003; Mrhalova et al., 2003; Dancey et al., 2003; Latif et al., 2004; Montemurro et al., 2004; Gatzemeier et al., 2004; Andre et al., 2004; Bianchi et al., 2003; Fuchs et al., 2003; Rowinsky, 2003; Barnes et al., 2002). For some monogenic diseases, patient numbers may be too small to support commercial development without changes to orphan drug legislation or payer willingness to accept higher cost-effectiveness thresholds. In the case of pharmacogenetics (Danzon et al., 2002), HER2 plays an important role in oncogenic transformation, tumorigenesis and metastatic spread. Clinical trials have also revealed several serious side-effects of monoclonal antibody therapy. Most notable is an unpredictable cardiotoxicity, especially when used in combination with anthracycline-based chemotherapy regimens (Leonard et al., 2002). This study sought to estimate cardiac dysfunction (CD) risk for patients receiving trastuzumab; to characterize treatment, and clinical outcome; to assess effects of baseline clinical risk factors on CD; and to assess effects of cumulative doses of anthracyclines and trastuzumab on CD (Baselga et al., 2002; Normanno et al., 2002). These data suggest that combined treatment with drugs that target HER2 might result in an efficient inhibition of tumor growth in those breast carcinoma patients whose tumors co-express both receptors (Zulkowski et al., 2002). In vitro assay, trastuzumab has been shown to inhibit the proliferation of human tumor cells that overexpressed HER2 and to be a mediator of antibody-dependent cellular toxicity. First-line trastuzumab in combination with chemotherapy, particularly paclitaxel, significantly improved time to disease progression, duration of response, and time to treatment failure (Hsu et al., 2002; Domenech et al., 2001). As combinations and sequences of anthracyclines and taxanes increasingly become standard Doublets or triplets of vinorelbine with drugs other than anthracyclines and taxanes could be considered in the next generation of adjuvant and neoadjuvant trials, where it is anticipated that anthracycline/taxane combinations are likely to replace anthracycline/cyclophosphamide combinations as the mainstay of adjuvant treatment (Ibrahim et al., 2001; Laufman et al., 2001; Martín, 2001). The clinical effectiveness of the other platinum compounds (iproplatin, oxaliplatin, and others) has not yet been fully tested as first-line chemotherapy. Cisplatin combinations have been employed as neoadjuvant chemotherapy in women with locally advanced breast cancer. The combinations of cisplatin with older pharmacological agents (5-fluorouracil, etoposide) have moderate activity, while the combinations of cisplatin with the newer agents (vinorelbine, paclitaxel, docetaxel, gemcitabine) appear to be more active. The combinations of carboplatin with the classical agents (5-fluorouracil, etoposide) are poorly active in previously treated MBC; Cisplatin, carboplatin, and perhaps, oxaliplatin appear to have some antitumor activity and can be combined safely with other agents that are active in this disease. However, the precise role that platinum compounds play in the treatment of breast cancer remains to be defined Sparano, 2000; (Krüger et al., 2002; Cardoso et al., 2002; Tan-Chiu et al., 2002; Le et al., 2003; Skálová et al., 2003; Heinemann, 2003; Vincent-Salomon et al., 2003; Cellini et al., 2002; Christodoulou et al., 2003; Horvai et al., 2003; Artemov et al., 2003; Bilous et al., 2003; (Clark et al., 2003; Penault-Llorca et al., 2002; Knowlden et al., 2003; O'Shaughnessy et al., 2003). The taxanes paclitaxel and docetaxel have an important role in the treatment of breast cancer, and numerous randomized trials have evaluated their efficacy for this indication (Robins et al., 2002; Cristofanilli et al., 2001). The management of metastatic breast cancer is changing as a consequence of extraordinary discoveries in cancer research and the development of more advanced diagnostic technologies. Although traditional chemotherapeutics such as anthracyclines and taxanes still represent the mainstay of treatment for this disease, new drugs are demonstrating significant clinical activity and sometimes a better toxicity profile. Furthermore, the successful introduction into clinical practice of biological agents, in particular the monoclonal antibody trastuzumab, offers a key to the future of managing metastatic breast cancer. A therapeutic approach based on modifications of a specific molecular target alone or combined with the traditional chemotherapeutic drugs is expected to be used more commonly bring significant improvement in the clinical response (Azzoli et al., 2002; (Eidtmann, 2002; Tulusan, 2002; Biganzoli et al., 2003; Miles et al., 2002; Besse et al., 2002; Van Poznak et al., 2002; Davidson, 2002; Nabholtz et al., 2002; Fornier et al., 2002). Despite intensive treatment efforts, the prognosis for lung cancer is very poor; less than 15% of patients survive 5 years. Trastuzumab, a monoclonal antibody targeting the HER2/neu protein receptor, is effective in the treatment of metastatic breast cancer and may be useful in the treatment of non-small cell lung cancer (NSCLC). Prospective clinical studies with trastuzumab in lung cancer are ongoing. Future studies in NSCLC need to include immunohistochemistry and fluorescence in situ hybridization analysis to determine the method of choice for evaluating clinically relevant HER2 positive tumors (Hirsch et al., 2002; Leslie et al., 2002; Runowicz et al.,

2001; Latif et al., 2002; Sorokin et al., 2002; (Perez et al., 2002; Kobayashi et al., 2002; Aikat et al., 2001; Bilous, 2001). Gemcitabine was identified as an active agent in the treatment of urothelial cancer early in its clinical development. A gemcitabine/cisplatin regimen has been shown to lead to comparable survival in a phase III comparison to methotrexate/ vinblastine/doxorubicin/cisplatin in the metastatic setting with less toxicity. Combinations with targeted therapeutic agents such as the epidermal growth factor receptor inhibitors and trastuzumab have great potential, but the clinical studies have not yet been completed (Stadler et al., 2002; Freebairn et al., 2001; Konecny et al., 2002; Hirsch et al., 2002; Fujimura et al., 2002; Hilfrich et al., 2002; von Minckwitz, 2002; Untch, 2002; Schaller, 2002; Meden, 2002). The main focus of the present study was to assess the efficacy of interphase cytogenetics using fluorescence in situ hybridization (FISH) as a valid alternative to immunohistochemistry (IHC) in paraffin-embedded tissue sections and/or the efficacy of the combination of the two methods, while, at the same time, aiming to provide additional information on the use of the two methods (Cianciulli et al., 2002; De Iuliis et al., 2017; Curigliano et al., 2017; Tran et al., 2017; Kim et al., 2017; Bozkurt et al., 2017; Hartmans et al., 2017; Lee et al., 2017; Tezuka et al., 2017; Bian et al., 2017; Zhou et al., 2017; Klein et al., 2017; Lopez-Albaitero et al., 2017; Ito et al., 2017; Ikink et al., 2017; Wagner-Rousset et al., 2017; Toi et al., 2017; Bianchi et al., 2003; Fuchs et al., 2003; Barnes et al., 2002). Short-term administration regimens yielding long-term therapeutic benefits are likely to meet payer resistance to large "one-off" costs because of budget constraints or, in competitive systems, concerns that the savings would accrue to future insurers or would attract high-cost patients. For some monogenic diseases, patient numbers may be too small to support commercial development without changes to orphan drug legislation or payer willingness to accept higher cost-effectiveness thresholds. Advances in molecular biology and improved understanding of tumour biology have led to the development of novel treatments for cancer. HER2 plays an important role in oncogenic transformation, tumorigenesis and metastatic spread. Overexpression is associated with a poor prognosis and predicts a poor response to several treatment modalities (Leonard et al., 2002; (Grossi et al., 2003; Goldman, 2003; Lu et al., 2004; Kauraniemi et al., 2004; Nihira, 2003; Aprikian et al., 2003; Urruticoechea et al., 2017; Kitayama et al., 2017; van Ramshorst et al., 2017; Zer et al., 2017). Trastuzumab is associated with an increased risk of CD, which is greatest in patients receiving concurrent anthracyclines. In most patients with metastatic breast cancer, the risk of CD can be justified given the improvement in overall survival previously reported with trastuzumab (Seidman et al., 2002).

ACKNOWLEDGMENTS

Dorota Bartusik-Aebisher acknowledges support from the National Center of Science NCN (New drug delivery systems-MRI study, Grant OPUS-13 number 2017/25/B/ST4/02481).

REFERENCES

Andre F, Le Chevalier T, Soria JC. Her2-neu: a target in lung cancer? *Ann Oncol.* 2004;15(1):3-4.

Artemov D, Mori N, Okollie B, Bhujwalla ZM. MR molecular imaging of the Her-2/neu receptor in breast cancer cells using targeted iron oxide nanoparticles. *Magn Reson Med.* 2003;49(3):403-8.

Azzoli CG, Krug LM, Miller VA, Kris MG, Mass R. Trastuzumab in the treatment of non-small cell lung cancer. *Semin Oncol.* 2002 Feb;29(1 Suppl 4):59-65. Review.

Bafaloukos D, Skarlos D. Weekly paclitaxel as first-line chemotherapy and trastuzumab in patients with advanced breast cancer. A Hellenic Cooperative Oncology Group phase II study. *Ann Oncol.* 2001;12(11):1545-51.

Barnes CJ, Li F, Mandal M, Yang Z, Sahin AA, Kumar R. Heregulin induces expression, ATPase activity, and nuclear localization of G3BP, a Ras signaling component, in human breast tumors. *Cancer Res.* 2002;62(5):1251-5.

Baselga J. Combined anti-EGF receptor and anti-HER2 receptor therapy in breast cancer: a promising strategy ready for clinical testing. *Ann Oncol.* 2002;13(1):8-9. No abstract available.

Besse B, Spano JP. Gemcitabine and breast cancer]. *Bull Cancer.* 2002;89 Spec No:S107-14.

Bian SX, Korah MP, Whitaker TR, Ji L, Groshen S, Chung E. No Acute Changes in LVEF Observed With Concurrent Trastuzumab and Breast Radiation With Low Heart Doses. *Clin Breast Cancer.* 2017; 17(7):510-515.

Bianchi G, Albanell J, Eiermann W, Vitali G, Borquez D, Viganò L, Molina R, Raab G, Locatelli A, Vanhauwere B, Gianni L, Baselga J. Pilot trial of trastuzumab starting with or after the doxorubicin component of a doxorubicin plus paclitaxel regimen for women with HER2-positive advanced breast cancer. *Clin Cancer Res.* 2003;9(16 Pt 1):5944-51.

Biganzoli L, Martin M, Twelves C. Moving forward with capecitabine: a glimpse of the future. Oncologist. 2002;7 Suppl 6:29-35. Review. Erratum in: *Oncologist.* 2003;8(1):127.

Bilous M, Dowsett M, Hanna W, Isola J, Lebeau A, Moreno A, Penault-Llorca F, Rüschoff J, Tomasic G, van de Vijver M. Current perspectives on HER2 testing: a review of national testing guidelines. *Mod Pathol.* 2003;16(2):173-82.

Bouchie A. Cancer trials get set for biomarkers. *Nat Biotechnol.* 2004;22(1):6-7. No abstract available. Erratum in: *Nat Biotechnol.* 2004;22(3):341.

Bozkurt M, Amlashi FG, Blum Murphy M. The role of chemotherapy in unresectable or metastatic adenocarcinoma of the stomach and gastroesophageal junction. *Minerva Chir.* 2017; 72(4):317-333.

Cardoso F, Piccart MJ, Durbecq V, Di Leo A. Resistance to trastuzumab: a necessary evil or a temporary challenge? *Clin Breast Cancer.* 2002;3(4):247-57; discussion 258-9.

Cellini N, Morganti AG, Macchia G, Smaniotto D, Luzi S, Mattiucci GC, Forni F, Valentini V. Biological factors and therapeutic modulation in pancreatic carcinoma radiotherapy. *Rays*. 2002;27(3):215-7.

Christodoulou C, Klouvas G, Pateli A, Mellou S, Sgouros J, Skarlos DV. Prolonged administration of weekly paclitaxel and trastuzumab in patients with advanced breast cancer. *Anticancer Res*. 2003;23(1B):737-44.

Cianciulli AM, Botti C, Coletta AM, Buglioni S, Marzano R, Benevolo M, Cione A, Mottolese M. Contribution of fluorescence in situ hybridization to immunohistochemistry for the evaluation of HER-2 in breast cancer. *Cancer Genet Cytogenet*. 2002;133(1):66-71.

Clark AS, West KA, Blumberg PM, Dennis PA. Altered protein kinase C (PKC) isoforms in non-small cell lung cancer cells: PKCdelta promotes cellular survival and chemotherapeutic resistance. *Cancer Res*. 2003;63(4):780-6.

Cobleigh M, Somberg JC. A case of herceptin cardiotoxicity. *Am J Ther*. 2004;11(1):74-6.

Cristofanilli M, Hortobagyi GN. New horizons in treating metastatic disease. *Clin Breast Cancer*. 2001;1(4):276-87.

Curigliano G, Goldhirsch A. Dual HER2 inhibition and pathological complete response in early breast cancer: increasing success of treatment by improving patient selection. *Ann Oncol*. 2017; 28(3):441-443.

Curigliano G, Goldhirsch A. Dual HER2 inhibition and pathological complete response in early breast cancer: increasing success of treatment by improving patient selection. *Ann Oncol*. 2017; 28(3):441-443.

Dancey JE. Recent advances of molecular targeted agents: opportunities for imaging. *Cancer Biol Ther*. 2003;2(6):601-9.

Danzon P, Towse A. The economics of gene therapy and of pharmacogenetics. *Value Health*. 2002;5(1):5-13.

Davidson NE. Ongoing US cooperative group trials using taxanes in the adjuvant setting. *Clin Breast Cancer*. 2002;3 Suppl 2:S53-8.

De Iuliis F, Salerno G, Taglieri L, Lanza R, Cardelli P, Scarpa S. Circulating neuregulin-1 and galectin-3 can be prognostic markers in breast cancer. *Int J Biol Markers*. 2017; 32(3):e333-e336.

De Iuliis F, Salerno G, Taglieri L, Lanza R, Cardelli P, Scarpa S. Circulating neuregulin-1 and galectin-3 can be prognostic markers in breast cancer. *Int J Biol Markers*. 2017; 32(3):e333-e336.

Domenech GH, Vogel CL. A review of vinorelbine in the treatment of breast cancer. *Clin Breast Cancer*. 2001;2(2):113-28.

Ebi H, Sasaki Y. [Rationale for Herceptin in the clinical use]. *Nihon Rinsho*. 2002;60(3):463-7.

Eidtmann H. [Herceptin monotherapy in HER2(+) recurrent breast carcinoma]. *Onkologie*. 2002;25 Suppl 5:14-5

Fornier M, Risio M, Van Poznak C, Seidman A. HER2 testing and correlation with efficacy of trastuzumab therapy. *Oncology* (Williston Park). 2002;16(10):1340-8.

Fuchs IB, Landt S, Bueler H, Kuehl U, Coupland S, Kleine-Tebbe A, Lichtenegger W, Schaller G. Analysis of HER2 and HER4 in human myocardium to clarify the cardiotoxicity of trastuzumab (Herceptin). *Breast Cancer Res Treat*. 2003;82(1):23-8.

Fuchs IB, Landt S, Bueler H, Kuehl U, Coupland S, Kleine-Tebbe A, Lichtenegger W, Schaller G. Analysis of HER2 and HER4 in human myocardium to clarify the cardiotoxicity of trastuzumab (Herceptin). *Breast Cancer Res Treat*. 2003;82(1):23-8.

Fujimura M, Katsumata N, Tsuda H, Uchi N, Miyazaki S, Hidaka T, Sakai M, Saito S. HER2 is frequently over-expressed in ovarian clear cell adenocarcinoma: possible novel treatment modality using recombinant monoclonal antibody against HER2, trastuzumab. *Jpn J Cancer Res*. 2002;93(11):1250-7.

Ganne C, Trillet-Lenoir V, Jaisson-Hot I, Chauvin F, Clippe C, Heilmann MO, Hajri T, Poncet B, Heuclin C, Colin C. [Which medico-economic approaches must be taken to evaluate the impact of costly molecules in oncology? The model of Herceptin in the breast metastatic cancer]. *Bull Cancer*. 2003;90(11):955-60.

Gatzemeier U, Groth G, Butts C, Van Zandwijk N, Shepherd F, Ardizzoni A, Barton C, Ghahramani P, Hirsh V. Randomized phase II trial of gemcitabine-cisplatin with or without trastuzumab in HER2-positive non-small-cell lung cancer. *Ann Oncol.* 2004;15(1):19-27.

Goldman B. For investigational targeted drugs, combination trials pose challenges. *J Natl Cancer Inst.* 2003;95(23):1744-6..

Goldman B. For investigational targeted drugs, combination trials pose challenges. *J Natl Cancer Inst.* 2003;95(23):1744-6.

Gori S, Colozza M, Mosconi AM, Franceschi E, Basurto C, Cherubini R, Sidoni A, Rulli A, Bisacci C, De Angelis V, Crinò L, Tonato M. Phase II study of weekly paclitaxel and trastuzumab in anthracycline and taxane-pretreated patients with HER2-overexpressing metastatic breast cancer. *Br J Cancer.* 2004;90(1):36-40.

Grossi PM, Ochiai H, Archer GE, McLendon RE, Zalutsky MR, Friedman AH, Friedman HS, Bigner DD, Sampson JH. Efficacy of intracerebral microinfusion of trastuzumab in an athymic rat model of intracerebral metastatic breast cancer. *Clin Cancer Res.* 2003;9(15):5514-20.

Grossi PM, Ochiai H, Archer GE, McLendon RE, Zalutsky MR, Friedman AH, Friedman HS, Bigner DD, Sampson JH. Efficacy of intracerebral microinfusion of trastuzumab in an athymic rat model of intracerebral metastatic breast cancer. *Clin Cancer Res.* 2003;9(15):5514-20.

Hartmans E, Linssen MD, Sikkens C, Levens A, Witjes MJH, van Dam GM, Nagengast WB. Tyrosine kinase inhibitor induced growth factor receptor upregulation enhances the efficacy of near-infrared targeted photodynamic therapy in esophageal adenocarcinoma cell lines. *Oncotarget.* 2017; 8(18):29846-29856.

Heinemann V. Role of gemcitabine in the treatment of advanced and metastatic breast cancer. *Oncology.* 2003;64(3):191-206.

Hilfrich J, Jänicke F. Therapy decision - patient participation?. *Onkologie.* 2002;25 Suppl 5:25-7.

Hirsch FR, Fischer JR, Niklinski J, Zöchbaüer-Müller S. Future developments in the treatment of lung cancer. *Lung Cancer.* 2002;38 Suppl 3:S81-5.

Hirsch FR, Franklin WA, Veve R, Varella-Garcia M, Bunn PA Jr. HER2/neu expression in malignant lung tumors. *Semin Oncol.* 2002;29(1 Suppl 4):51-8.

Horvai AE, Li L, Xu Z, Kramer MJ, Jablons DM, Treseler PA. Malignant mesothelioma does not demonstrate overexpression or gene amplification despite cytoplasmic immunohistochemical staining for c-Erb-B2. *Arch Pathol Lab Med.* 2003;127(4):465-9.

Hsu C, Huang CL, Hsu HC, Lee PH, Wang SJ, Cheng AL. HER-2/neu overexpression is rare in hepatocellular carcinoma and not predictive of anti-HER-2/neu regulation of cell growth and chemosensitivity. *Cancer.* 2002;94(2):415-20.

Ibrahim NK. Commentary on "A review of vinorelbine in the treatment of breast cancer." *Clin Breast Cancer.* 2001;2(3):236.

Ikink GJ, Hilkens J. Insulin receptor substrate 4 (IRS4) is a constitutive active oncogenic driver collaborating with HER2 and causing therapeutic resistance. *Mol Cell Oncol.* 2017; 4(2):e1279722.

Ito K, Mitsunaga M, Nishimura T, Saruta M, Iwamoto T, Kobayashi H, Tajiri H. Near-Infrared Photochemoimmunotherapy by Photo-activatable Bifunctional Antibody-Drug Conjugates Targeting Human Epidermal Growth Factor Receptor 2 Positive Cancer. *Bioconjug Chem.* 2017; 28(5):1458-1469.

Kauraniemi P, Hautaniemi S, Autio R, Astola J, Monni O, Elkahloun A, Kallioniemi A. Effects of Herceptin treatment on global gene expression patterns in HER2-amplified and nonamplified breast cancer cell lines. *Oncogene.* 2004;23(4):1010-3.

Kauraniemi P, Hautaniemi S, Autio R, Astola J, Monni O, Elkahloun A, Kallioniemi A. Effects of Herceptin treatment on global gene expression patterns in HER2-amplified and nonamplified breast cancer cell lines. *Oncogene.* 2004;23(4):1010-3.

Kim HS, Lee H, Shin SJ, Beom SH, Jung M, Bae S, Lee EY, Park KH, Choi YY, Son T, Kim HI, Cheong JH, Hyung WJ, Park JC, Shin SK, Lee SK, Lee YC, Koom WS, Lim JS, Chung HC, Noh SH, Rha SY, Kim H, Paik S. Complementary utility of targeted next-generation sequencing and immunohistochemistry panels as a screening platform to select targeted therapy for advanced gastric cancer. *Oncotarget.* 2017; 8(24):38389-38398.

Kitayama H, Kondo T, Sugiyama J, Kurimoto K, Nishino Y, Kawada M, Hirayama M, Tsuji Y. High-sensitive troponin T assay can predict anthracycline- and trastuzumab-induced cardiotoxicity in breast cancer patients. *Breast Cancer.* 2017; 24(6):774-782.

Kitayama H, Kondo T, Sugiyama J, Kurimoto K, Nishino Y, Kawada M, Hirayama M, Tsuji Y. High-sensitive troponin T assay can predict anthracycline- and trastuzumab-induced cardiotoxicity in breast cancer patients. *Breast Cancer.* 2017; 24(6):774-782.

Klein C, Waldhauer I, Nicolini VG, Freimoser-Grundschober A, Nayak T, Vugts DJ, Dunn C, Bolijn M, Benz J, Stihle M, Lang S, Roemmele M, Hofer T, van Puijenbroek E, Wittig D, Moser S, Ast O, Brünker P, Gorr IH, Neumann S, de Vera Mudry MC, Hinton H, Crameri F, Saro J, Evers S, Gerdes C, Bacac M, van Dongen G, Moessner E, Umaña P. Cergutuzumab amunaleukin (CEA-IL2v), a CEA-targeted IL-2 variant-based immunocytokine for combination cancer immunotherapy: Overcoming limitations of aldesleukin and conventional IL-2-based immunocytokines. *Oncoimmunology.* 2017; 6(3):e1277306.

Knowlden JM, Hutcheson IR, Jones HE, Madden T, Gee JM, Harper ME, Barrow D, Wakeling AE, Nicholson RI. Elevated levels of epidermal growth factor receptor/c-erbB2 heterodimers mediate an autocrine growth regulatory pathway in tamoxifen-resistant MCF-7 cells. *Endocrinology.* 2003;144(3):1032-44.

Konecny G, Slamon DJ. HER2 testing and correlation with efficacy of trastuzumab therapy. *Oncology* (Williston Park). 2002;16(11):1576, 1578.

Krüger S, Weitsch G, Büttner H, Matthiensen A, Böhmer T, Marquardt T, Sayk F, Feller AC, Böhle A. HER2 overexpression in muscle-invasive urothelial carcinoma of the bladder: prognostic implications. *Int J Cancer.* 2002;102(5):514-8.

Kubo M, Morisaki T, Kuroki H, Tasaki A, Yamanaka N, Matsumoto K, Nakamura K, Onishi H, Baba E, Katano M. Combination of adoptive immunotherapy with Herceptin for patients with HER2-expressing breast cancer. *Anticancer Res.* 2003;23(6a):4443-9.

Kubo M, Morisaki T, Kuroki H, Tasaki A, Yamanaka N, Matsumoto K, Nakamura K, Onishi H, Baba E, Katano M. Combination of adoptive immunotherapy with Herceptin for patients with HER2-expressing breast cancer. *Anticancer Res.* 2003;23(6a):4443-9.

Latif Z, Watters AD, Dunn I, Grigor K, Underwood MA, Bartlett JM. HER2/neu gene amplification and protein overexpression in G3 pT2 transitional cell carcinoma of the bladder: a role for anti-HER2 therapy? *Eur J Cancer.* 2004;40(1):56-63.

Laufman LR, Forsthoefel KF. Use of intrathecal trastuzumab in a patient with carcinomatous meningitis. *Clin Breast Cancer.* 2001;2(3):235.

Le XF, Claret FX, Lammayot A, Tian L, Deshpande D, LaPushin R, Tari AM, Bast RC Jr. The role of cyclin-dependent kinase inhibitor p27Kip1 in anti-HER2 antibody-induced G1 cell cycle arrest and tumor growth inhibition. *J Biol Chem.* 2003;278(26):23441-50.

Lee CK, Kim SS, Park S, Kim C, Heo SJ, Lim JS, Kim H, Kim HS, Rha SY, Chung HC, Park S, Jung M. Depth of response is a significant predictor for long-term outcome in advanced gastric cancer patients treated with trastuzumab. *Oncotarget.* 2017; 8(19):31169-31179.

Leonard DS, Hill AD, Kelly L, Dijkstra B, McDermott E, O'Higgins NJ. Anti-human epidermal growth factor receptor 2 monoclonal antibody therapy for breast cancer. *Br J Surg.* 2002;89(3):262-71.

Leyland-Jones B. Trastuzumab: hopes and realities. *Lancet Oncol.* 2002;3(3):137-44.

Lopez-Albaitero A, Xu H, Guo H, Wang L, Wu Z, Tran H, Chandarlapaty S, Scaltriti M, Janjigian Y, de Stanchina E, Cheung NK. Overcoming resistance to HER2-targeted therapy with a novel HER2/CD3 bispecific antibody. *Oncoimmunology.* 2017; 6(3):e1267891.

Lu Y, Zi X, Pollak M. Molecular mechanisms underlying IGF-I-induced attenuation of the growth-inhibitory activity of trastuzumab (Herceptin) on SKBR3 breast cancer cells. *Int J Cancer.* 2004 20;108(3):334-41.

Lu Y, Zi X, Pollak M. Molecular mechanisms underlying IGF-I-induced attenuation of the growth-inhibitory activity of trastuzumab (Herceptin) on SKBR3 breast cancer cells. *Int J Cancer*. 2004;108(3): 334-41.

Lu Y, Zi X, Zhao Y, Pollak M. Overexpression of ErbB2 receptor inhibits IGF-I-induced Shc-MAPK signaling pathway in breast cancer cells. *Biochem Biophys Res Commun*. 2004;313(3):709-15.

Martín M. Platinum compounds in the treatment of advanced breast cancer. *Clin Breast Cancer*. 2001;2(3):190-208.

Meden H. Combination therapy herceptin+taxotere/Herceptin+navelbine. *Onkologie*. 2002;25 Suppl 5:15-6.

Miles D, von Minckwitz G, Seidman AD. Combination versus sequential single-agent therapy in metastatic breast cancer. *Oncologist*. 2002;7 Suppl 6:13-9.

Montemurro F, Valabrega G, Aglietta M. Trastuzumab-based combination therapy for breast cancer. *Expert Opin Pharmacother*. 2004;5(1):81-96.

Mrhalova M, Kodet R. Paget's disease of the nipple: a copy number of the genes ERBB2 and CCND1 versus expression of the proteins ERBB-2 and cyclin D1. *Neoplasma*. 2003;50(6):396-402.

Nabholtz JM, Reese DM, Lindsay MA, Riva A. HER2-positive breast cancer: update on Breast Cancer International Research Group trials. *Clin Breast Cancer*. 2002;3 Suppl 2:S75-9.

Nihira S. Development of HER2-specific humanized antibody Herceptin (trastuzumab). *Nihon Yakurigaku Zasshi*. 2003;122(6):504-14.

Nihira S. Development of HER2-specific humanized antibody Herceptin (trastuzumab). *Nihon Yakurigaku Zasshi*. 2003;122(6):504-14.

Normanno N, Campiglio M, De LA, Somenzi G, Maiello M, Ciardiello F, Gianni L, Salomon DS, Menard S. Cooperative inhibitory effect of ZD1839 (Iressa) in combination with trastuzumab (Herceptin) on human breast cancer cell growth. *Ann Oncol*. 2002; 13(1):65-72.

O'Shaughnessy JA. Pegylated liposomal doxorubicin in the treatment of breast cancer. *Clin Breast Cancer*. 2003;4(5):318-28.

Penault-Llorca F, Etessami A, Bourhis J. [Principal therapeutic uses of monoclonal antibodies in oncology]. *Cancer Radiother.* 2002;6 Suppl 1:24s-28s.

Rivera E. Current status of liposomal anthracycline therapy in metastatic breast cancer. *Clin Breast Cancer.* 2003 Suppl 2:S76-83.

Rivera E. Current status of liposomal anthracycline therapy in metastatic breast cancer. *Clin Breast Cancer.* 2003;4 Suppl 2:S76-83.

Robins HI, Liu G, Hayes L, Mehta M. Trastuzumab for breast cancer-related carcinomatous meningitis. *Clin Breast Cancer.* 2002;2(4):316.

Ross JS, Gray GS. Targeted therapy for cancer: the HER-2/neu and Herceptin story. *Clin Leadersh Manag Rev.* 2003;17(6):333-40.

Rowinsky EK. Signal events: Cell signal transduction and its inhibition in cancer. *Oncologist.* 2003;8 Suppl 3:5-17.

Rowinsky EK. Signal events: Cell signal transduction and its inhibition in cancer. *Oncologist.* 2003;8 Suppl 3:5-17.

Schaller G. Combination therapy herceptin+xeloda]. *Onkologie.* 2002;25 Suppl 5:17-8.

Seidman A, Hudis C, Pierri MK, Shak S, Paton V, Ashby M, Murphy M, Stewart SJ, Keefe D. Cardiac dysfunction in the trastuzumab clinical trials experience. *J Clin Oncol.* 2002;20(5):1215-21.

Skálová A, Vaněcek T, Losan F, Papoutsidesová, Fínek J. [Detection of HER-2/neu in breast carcinoma]. *Cas Lek Cesk.* 2003;142(2):93-8. Czech.

Sledge GW Jr. The HERstory of breast cancer revealed. *Clin Breast Cancer.* 2003;4(5):308. No abstract available.

Sparano JA. Taxanes for breast cancer: an evidence-based review of randomized phase II and phase III trials. *Clin Breast Cancer.* 2000;1(1):32-40.

Speyer J. Cardiac dysfunction in the trastuzumab clinical experience. *J Clin Oncol.* 2002 Mar 1;20(5):1156-7. No abstract available.

Stadler WM. Gemcitabine doublets in advanced urothelial cancer. *Semin Oncol.* 2002;29(1 Suppl 3):15-9.

Sun Y, Li LQ, Song ST, Xu LG, Yu SY, Wang JW, Jiang ZF, Yin JL, Xiong HH. Result of phase II clinical trial of herceptin in advanced

Chinese breast cancer patients. *Zhonghua Zhong Liu Za Zhi.* 2003 Nov;25(6):581-3.

Tan-Chiu E, Piccart M. Moving forward: Herceptin in the adjuvant setting. *Oncology.* 2002;63 Suppl 1:57-63.

Tezuka K, Takashima T, Kashiwagi S, Kawajiri H, Tokunaga S, Tei S, Nishimura S, Yamagata S, Noda S, Nishimori T, Mizuyama Y, Sunami T, Ikeda K, Ogawa Y, Onoda N, Ishikawa T, Kudoh S, Takada M, Hirakawa K. Phase I study of nanoparticle albumin-bound paclitaxel, carboplatin and trastuzumab in women with human epidermal growth factor receptor 2-overexpressing breast cancer. *Mol Clin Oncol.* 2017; 6(4):534-538.

Theodoulou M, Seidman AD. Cardiac effects of adjuvant therapy for early breast cancer. *Semin Oncol.* 2003;30(6):730-9.

Theodoulou M, Seidman AD. Cardiac effects of adjuvant therapy for early breast cancer. *Semin Oncol.* 2003;30(6):730-9.

Toi M, Shao Z, Hurvitz S, Tseng LM, Zhang Q, Shen K, Liu D, Feng J, Xu B, Wang X, Lee KS, Ng TY, Ridolfi A, Noel-Baron F, Ringeisen F, Jiang Z. Efficacy and safety of everolimus in combination with trastuzumab and paclitaxel in Asian patients with HER2+ advanced breast cancer in BOLERO-1. *Breast Cancer Res.* 2017; 19(1):47.

Tokuda Y, Saito Y, Suzuki Y, Ohta M, Tajima T. [Breast cancer]. *Nihon Rinsho.* 2002;60(3):563-9.

Tran WT, Gangeh MJ, Sannachi L, Chin L, Watkins E, Bruni SG, Rastegar RF, Curpen B, Trudeau M, Gandhi S, Yaffe M, Slodkowska E, Childs C, Sadeghi-Naini A, Czarnota GJ. Predicting breast cancer response to neoadjuvant chemotherapy using pretreatment diffuse optical spectroscopic texture analysis. *Br J Cancer.* 2017; 116(10):1329-1339.

Tran WT, Gangeh MJ, Sannachi L, Chin L, Watkins E, Bruni SG, Rastegar RF, Curpen B, Trudeau M, Gandhi S, Yaffe M, Slodkowska E, Childs C, Sadeghi-Naini A, Czarnota GJ. Predicting breast cancer response to neoadjuvant chemotherapy using pretreatment diffuse optical spectroscopic texture analysis. *Br J Cancer.* 2017; 116(10):1329-1339.

Tulusan AH. [DCIS and HER2/neu]. *Onkologie.* 2002;25 Suppl 5:11-2.

Untch M. [Therapy concept: herceptin with anthracyclines]. *Onkologie.* 2002;25 Suppl 5:19-21.

Urruticoechea A, Rizwanullah M, Im SA, Ruiz ACS, Láng I, Tomasello G, Douthwaite H, Badovinac Crnjevic T, Heeson S, Eng-Wong J, Muñoz M. Randomized Phase III Trial of Trastuzumab Plus Capecitabine With or Without Pertuzumab in Patients With Human Epidermal Growth Factor Receptor 2-Positive Metastatic Breast Cancer Who Experienced Disease Progression During or After Trastuzumab-Based Therapy. *J Clin Oncol.* 2017; 35(26):3030-3038.

Urruticoechea A, Rizwanullah M, Im SA, Ruiz ACS, Láng I, Tomasello G, Douthwaite H, Badovinac Crnjevic T, Heeson S, Eng-Wong J, Muñoz M. Randomized Phase III Trial of Trastuzumab Plus Capecitabine With or Without Pertuzumab in Patients With Human Epidermal Growth Factor Receptor 2-Positive Metastatic Breast Cancer Who Experienced Disease Progression During or After Trastuzumab-Based Therapy. *J Clin Oncol.* 2017; 35(26):3030-3038.

Van Poznak C, Seidman AD. Critical review of current treatment strategies for advanced hormone insensitive breast cancer. *Cancer Invest.* 2002;20 Suppl 2:1-14.

van Ramshorst MS, Loo CE, Groen EJ, Winter-Warnars GH, Wesseling J, van Duijnhoven F, Peeters MTV, Sonke GS. MRI predicts pathologic complete response in HER2-positive breast cancer after neoadjuvant chemotherapy. *Breast Cancer Res Treat.* 2017; 164(1):99-106.

van Ramshorst MS, Loo CE, Groen EJ, Winter-Warnars GH, Wesseling J, van Duijnhoven F, Peeters MTV, Sonke GS. MRI predicts pathologic complete response in HER2-positive breast cancer after neoadjuvant chemotherapy. *Breast Cancer Res Treat.* 2017; 164(1):99-106.

van Zanten J, Doornbos-Van der Meer B, Audouy S, Kok RJ, de Leij L. A nonviral carrier for targeted gene delivery to tumor cells. *Cancer Gene Ther.* 2004;11(2):156-64.

Vincent-Salomon A, MacGrogan G, Couturier J, Arnould L, Mathoulin-Pélissier S; Groupe d'Etude des Facteurs Pronostiques par Immunohistochime dans les Cancers du Sein. HER2 testing in the real world. *J Natl Cancer Inst.* 2003;95(8):628.

von Minckwitz G. Therapy concept: herceptin in combination with arimidex. *Onkologie*. 2002;25 Suppl 5:22.

Wagner-Rousset E, Fekete S, Morel-Chevillet L, Colas O, Corvaïa N, Cianférani S, Guillarme D, Beck A. Development of a fast workflow to screen the charge variants of therapeutic antibodies. *J Chromatogr A*. 2017; 1498:147-154.

Zer C, Avery KN, Meyer K, Goodstein L, Bzymek KP, Singh G, Williams JC. Engineering a high-affinity peptide binding site into the anti-CEA mAb M5A. *Protein Eng Des Sel*. 2017; 30(6):409-417.

Zhou Z, Vaidyanathan G, McDougald D, Kang CM, Balyasnikova I, Devoogdt N, Ta AN, McNaughton BR, Zalutsky MR. Fluorine-18 Labeling of the HER2-Targeting Single-Domain Antibody 2Rs15d Using a Residualizing Label and Preclinical Evaluation. *Mol Imaging Biol*. 2017; 19(6):867-877.

Zulkowski K, Kath R, Semrau R, Merkle K, Höffken K. Regression of brain metastases from breast carcinoma after chemotherapy with bendamustine. *J Cancer Res Clin Oncol*. 2002;128(2):111-3.

Chapter 3

TRASTUZUMAB: PHARMACODYNAMIC PROPERTIES

ABSTRACT

Trastuzumab is a recombinant humanized IgG1 monoclonal antibody. Overexpression of HER2 is observed in 20%-30% of primary breast cancers, gastric cancer (GC) using immunohistochemistry (IHC) and fluorescence in situ hybridization (FISH) or chromogenic in situ hybridization (CISH) have shown that there is a broad variation of HER2-positivity. In this chapter pharmacodynamic properties of Trastuzmab will be discussed.

Keywords: trastuzmab, pharmacodynamic properties, breast cancers, gastric cancer

Currently, immunohistochemistry and fluorescence in situ hybridization are the main tests used for HER2 detection (Bilous, 2001). Trastuzumab is the first monoclonal antibody to be approved for the treatment of a solid tumors and is directed against the c-erb-B2 receptor (Freebairn et al., 2001). To evaluate amplification of the HER-2 gene by fluorescence in situ hybridization (FISH) in tumors is recommend (Zulkowski et al., 2002; Leslie et al., 2002; Runowicz et al., 2001; Latif et al., 2002; Sorokin et al., 2000; Perez et al., 2002; Kobayashi et al., 2002).

Trastuzumab has ushered in hope for thousands of women, but its use mandates that a clear understanding of its effects and relative risks be appreciated (Aikat et al., 2001). Clinical trials with trastuzumab, a humanized anti-p185 HER-2/neu monoclonal antibody have demonstrated that this agent produces objective responses in patients with breast cancer. The combination of weekly paclitaxel and trastuzumab is a safe and active regimen for patients with HER-2/neu overexpressing ABC (Fountzilas et al., 2001; Vogel et al., 2002). The tumor antigen HER2 belongs to the epidermal growth factor receptor family. Numerous studies have shown that HER2 is overexpressed in many cancers and it is prognostically important in a subset of malignancies (Yip et al., 2002; Susnjar et al., 2001; Umemura et al., 2001). Appropriate evaluations of biological markers are essential for targeting therapy (Umemura et al., 2001). The HER-2 protein is thought to be a unique and useful target for antibody therapy of cancers overexpressing HER-2 (Tokuda et al., 2001). Binding with high affinity to the extracellular domain of HER2, trastuzumab inhibits the proliferation of tumor cells that overexpress HER2. A large well designed multicenter study found that the addition of trastuzumab to either an anthracycline plus cyclophosphamide or to paclitaxel, as first-line therapy for metastatic breast cancer overexpressing the HER2 receptor, significantly increased time to disease progression, rate of objective response, duration of response and survival compared with chemotherapy alone. Single-agent trastuzumab was associated with an objective response in 15% of extensively pretreated patients with metastatic breast cancer overexpressing HER2, and 26% of previously untreated patients. Trastuzumab has demonstrated synergistic action with several chemotherapy agents preclinically, but the optimal combination clinically is yet to be determined. Trastuzumab is generally well tolerated by most patients; the most significant adverse effects being acute fever and/or chills and the potential to cause cardiac dysfunction. Serious adverse events, including anaphylaxis and death, have occurred in 0.25% of patients. Symptomatic or asymptomatic cardiac dysfunction occurred in 13% of patients receiving trastuzumab plus paclitaxel and in 4.7% of patients receiving trastuzumab alone. Intravenous trastuzumab is effective as a single-agent, and in combination with chemotherapy it significantly improves the median time to disease progression and survival time in patients with metastatic breast cancer overexpressing the HER2 receptor compared with chemotherapy alone. Cardiotoxicity is the main concern with therapy; particularly in patients with pre-existing cardiac dysfunction, the elderly and in combination with, or following, anthracyclines. Trastuzumab is indicated for use with paclitaxel as first-line therapy or as a single agent in second- or third-line treatment regimens for patients with metastatic breast cancer overexpressing HER2. Investigation is ongoing to ascertain the optimal combination regimen containing trastuzumab and antineoplastic agents. In addition, current research is focusing on the optimal timing, sequencing and duration of therapy as well as administration in the neoadjuvant and adjuvant setting (McKeage et al., 2002; Savinainen et al., 2002). HER2/neu amplification/overexpression confers more aggressive and malignant characteristics on breast cancer cells. Patients with HER2/neu-amplified breast cancer have a worse prognosis than those with normal HER2/neu expression. Over the past decade, the intracellular signaling pathways associated with this growth factor receptor have been elucidated. In addition, when added to chemotherapy, trastuzumab improves antitumor efficacy as measured by time to progression, response rate, and survival. Additional chemotherapy/trastuzumab combinations are under active evaluation, and new schedules of administration are being tested. Thus, trastuzumab is the first successful example of molecularly targeted therapy in the management of metastatic breast cancer (Hortobagyi et al., 2001). Signaling by the HER2 proto-oncogene product results in the activation of several biochemical pathways that in turn modulate the expression and function of molecules involved in cell proliferation and survival. It is well established that forced overexpression of HER2 results in transformation of non-tumor cells, and that high levels of HER2 in tumors are associated with a more aggressive biological behavior. Over the last few years, several elegant studies have dissected the biochemical mechanisms of HER2 signaling. This research has provided information about critical functional domains in HER2 that can be targeted with rational molecular approaches, some of which are already being implemented at the bedside (Arteaga et al., 2001). Expression of these transcriptional regulators resulted in downregulation of HER2/neu promoter activity and reversed the transformed phenotype of the cancer cells in vitro. In vivo studies show that these HER2/neu repressors can act therapeutically as tumor suppressor genes for tumors that overexpress HER2/neu (Wang et al., 2001). HER2 is a transmembrane growth factor receptor found in normal and malignant breast epithelial cells. Phosphorylation of the intracellular tyrosine kinase results in intracellular signaling and activation of genes involved in cell growth. Prospective stratification of HER2 status in current clinical trials may more accurately delineate these roles. A potential limitation to its use in the adjuvant setting is the increased incidence of cardiotoxicity in patients treated either concurrently or previously with anthracyclines (Lohrisch et al., 2001). HER-2 has a well-established role as a prognostic indicator in breast cancer and as a predictor for response to trastuzumab. This article argues that the data are insufficient to accept this hypothesis as scientifically established. The argument is developed along several lines: first, that the trials used to support a predictive role for HER-2 have real flaws with regard to this hypothesis; second, that HER-2 is a remarkably inconsistent predictor of anthracycline response when examined in a broader context that includes preoperative and metastatic disease; third, that preclinical data fail to support the hypothesis; and finally, that even if accepted, the hypothesis is difficult to extrapolate to the everyday world of breast cancer (Sledge et al., 2001; (Wood et al., 2001). The metastatic lesion decreased in size and finally appeared to be only cicatricial. The pathological examination revealed no tumor cells in the resected specimen so further treatment was stopped. The relapse-free state has continued for 24 months after the pulmonary resection (Ohta et al., 2001). The HER2 protein is encoded by the HER2/neu gene and it is homologous to the epidermal growth factor receptor. Overexpression of HER2, usually in association with gene amplification, occurs in approximately 25-30% of breast cancers. The HER2 protein is a viable therapeutic target. The humanized anti-HER2 monoclonal antibody trastuzumab has demonstrated activity in clinical trials in women with metastatic breast cancer overexpressing HER2. The mechanisms of the action of this antibody involve disruption of DNA repair and induction of antibody-dependent cellular cytotoxicity. Response rates to the antibody given as a single agent in the treatment of HER2 overexpressing metastatic breast cancer have ranged from 12 to 27%. Patients who received trastuzumab in combination with chemotherapy had a significantly longer time to progression, higher overall survival compared with patients who had received chemotherapy alone. Trastuzumab has an important role in the treatment of HER2 overexpressing metastatic breast cancer. Its place in adjuvant treatment has not been proved up to now. The optimal use of trastuzumab in the treatment of HER2 positive advanced breast cancer is under active investigation. Due to the high rate of clinical activity and low incidence of severe toxicity trastuzumab is a very promising drug in the treatment of breast cancer. The author's purpose was to summarize the results of the trials using trastuzumab treatment, and discuss the methods used to determine the HER2 status (Dank et al., 2001). Herceptin is a humanized antibody that binds to the product of the HER-2 oncogene. Four different cell lines were used that had different levels of HER-2 expression. This effect is a decrease in cell proliferation that is coincident with, and may be caused by an increase frequency of DNA strand breaks (Mayfield et al., 2001). HER2 overexpression in breast cancer is associated with a poor prognosis, resistance to endocrine therapy and chemosensitivity to anthracyclines and paclitaxel. Moreover, trastuzumab shows therapeutic benefit in patients with HER2 overexpressing tumors. In addition to a definitive histological diagnosis, core biopsies of tumors offer the opportunity to evaluate the HER2 status (Mueller-Holzner et al., 2001). Data from phase III clinical trials suggest that high dose chemotherapy (HDC) is currently not indicated for any stage of breast cancer. Furthermore, there is no significant evidence to support the routine use of taxanes in women with metastatic breast cancer and further research is required to address this issue. A well-designed randomized controlled trial has shown that expressive support psychosocial therapy does not improve survival of women with MBC. Biological therapy using inhibitors/ antagonists of angiogenesis and EGFR seems to be safe and well tolerated.

Although the response rates are currently unimpressive, further research using survival as an endpoint is required (Mokbel et al., 2001). Development of resistance to trastuzumab, however, is common (Lu et al., 2001; Albanell et al., 2001; Moulder et al., 2001). ErbB-2 is ubiquitinated and degraded when dissociated from its membrane chaperone or bound by specific antibody. Reagents which induce such degradation have demonstrated antitumor activity and may impact ErbB-2 immunogenicity (Piechocki et al., 2001). Overexpression of HER-2) oncoprotein is an important prognostic factor associated with a poor prognosis in breast cancer. Although treatment with trastuzumab, an anti-HER-2 antibody, increases drug-sensitivity in vitro and in vivo, the role of HER-2 oncoprotein in drug-sensitivity is still uncertain. The present work discusses the clinical significance of the HER-2 oncoprotein in drug-sensitivity in breast cancer based on previous clinical and basic results and reviews the current concept of HER-2 oncoprotein in drug-sensitivity. Introduction of HER-2 oncoprotein in vitro induces resistance to several anticancer drugs, including taxanes, cisplatin and 5-fluorouracil in breast cancer cells. The acquisition of drug-resistance by introduction of the HER2 gene, however, depends on the cell type, because transfection of the HER2 gene per se does not necessarily induce resistance to the same drugs in all types of breast cancer cells. In clinical studies, patients with HER-2 overexpression responded better to an anthracycline-based regimen than patients with low HER-2 expression, and their overall survival was also superior. Taxanes responsiveness in patients with HER-2 oncoprotein overexpression was superior in patients with low HER2 expression (Kim et al., 2002). Herceptin is the first therapy for breast cancer which targets an oncogene product. Use of herceptin as a first-line therapy for metastatic disease in early studies suggests that response rates and clinical benefit rate similar to chemotherapy may be achievable and that survival using this sequential approach may not be compromised. The non-linear pharmacokinetics of herceptin suggests that, as doses increased half-life increases and may be feasible on a 3-weekly schedule. The role of herceptin in the adjuvant setting in the management of breast cancer will be tested in randomized studies of patients who express HER2 at the highest levels; two of these studies have already begun (Miles et al., 2001). The anthracycline antibiotic doxorubicin has wide activity against a number of human neoplasms and is used extensively both as a single agent and in combination regimens. One of the key toxicity issues linked to the use of free doxorubicin is that of both an acute and a chronic form of cardiomyopathy. This is circumvented by the use of liposomal formulations, as these systems tend to sequester the drug away from organs such as the heart, with greater accumulation in liver, spleen and tumors. However, as will be discussed, the liposomal formulations of doxorubicin are not without their own related toxicities, and, in the case of Doxil, may be associated with the unique toxicity of palmar-plantar erythrodysaesthesia (Waterhouse et al., 2001). In the future, in addition to targeting a patient's drug concentrations within a therapeutic range, pharmacists are likely to be making dosage recommendations for individual drugs on the basis of the individual patient's genotype (Ensom et al., 2001). A key target being actively pursued is the receptor tyrosine kinase. Several compounds that inhibit this target are in preclinical and clinical development. These compounds broadly fall into two categories: monoclonal antibodies and small-molecule inhibitors. Other uses are being tested, such as imatinib for gastrointestinal stromal tumor. These compounds will alter cancer care as adjuncts to currently available treatment options (Goel et al., 2001). Over the past decade, the clinical utility of monoclonal antibodies has been realized and antibodies are now a mainstay for the treatment of cancer. This multifaceted mechanism of action combined with target specificity underlies the capacity of antibodies to elicit anti-tumor responses while minimizing the frequency and magnitude of adverse events. This review will focus on mechanisms of action, clinical applications and putative mechanisms of resistance to monoclonal antibody therapy in the context of cancer (Crown et al., 2001), Hehl et al., 2001). Trastuzumab resulted in a complete and long-lasting response of recurrent and locally advanced breast cancer and was well tolerated in a severely cytotoxically pretreated patient with cardiac failure. (Hehl et al., 2001). Several agents that target one or more members of the erbB family of receptor tyrosine kinases are currently undergoing clinical investigation (Slichenmyer et al., 2001). Clinical trials using the humanized version of the anti-HER2 murine monoclonal antibody 4D5, trastuzumab, have shown antitumor activity in patients with HER2-positive metastatic breast cancer. Improved response and survival rates have been shown when trastuzumab was added to first-line combination chemotherapy with anthracycline/cyclophosphamide or paclitaxel compared with the same chemotherapy alone. Because of the promising safety and efficacy profile of trastuzumab in the metastatic setting, this novel biologic has now entered adjuvant breast cancer trials in both the United States and Europe. Five clinical trials are discussed in this report, capturing the evolving role of trastuzumab as adjuvant therapy for breast cancer (Hortobagyi et al., 2001). A full understanding of the mechanisms not only of antitumor activity but also of side effects and toxicity is critical to select the optimal schedule of administration. In this regard, preclinical (in vitro and in vivo) studies are often helpful before clinical studies are initiated. However, no preclinical model is fully predictive of the outcome of human clinical trials. Therefore, while preclinical studies can point to potentially fruitful directions in clinical investigation, only after fairly substantial clinical experience does the medical community reach agreement and understanding of the optimal dose and schedule of administration of an agent. For some agents, these conclusions are reached early in the development of the drug (eg, cyclophosphamide, docetaxel). For others (eg, fluorouracil, cytosine arabinoside) the definition of optimal dose and schedule of administration is a never-ending story. The optimal duration of administration for trastuzumab is not known and is currently under active investigation. Recent studies have established that growth factors and their receptors play an essential role in regulating the proliferation of epithelial cells. Abnormalities in the expression, structure, or activity of their proto-oncogene products contribute to the development and maintenance of the malignant phenotype. Tumor cells must use the process of vascularization (angiogenesis) for productive growth and metastasis. Overexpression of HER2 in human tumor cells is closely associated with increased angiogenesis and expression of vascular endothelial growth factor (VEGF). The anti-HER2 blocking antibody trastuzumab has been shown to inhibit tumor cell growth and VEGF expression. Cancer cell invasiveness can be promoted, even in the absence of HER2 overexpression, by transregulation of HER2 by heregulins that bind to HER3 and HER4. Accordingly, heregulin beta1 regulates the expression and secretion of VEGF in breast cancer cells, and trastuzumab inhibits heregulin-mediated angiogenesis both in vitro and in vivo. Thus, potential upregulation of VEGF in cancer epithelial cells likely supports angiogenesis, sustaining and promoting survival and metastasis of tumor cells (Kumar et al., 2001). Cardiotoxicity is a common and potentially devastating side effect of antineoplastic drug therapy. This empiric observation is seen as paradoxical given that the cardiomyocyte is considered to be a terminally differentiated cell. Trastuzumab/ anthracycline cardiomyopathy may be the first clinically significant cardiotoxicity to emerge from signal transduction therapeutics. Most importantly, these data draw attention to the inherent risk of cardiotoxicity associated with a newly emerging class of antineoplastic drugs that interfere with signal transduction pathways (Schneider et al., 2001). One of the molecular mechanisms of ErbB2-mediated paclitaxel resistance is that overexpression of the ErbB2 receptor leads to deregulation of the G2/M cell cycle check-point that inhibits paclitaxel-induced apoptosis. Several promising ErbB2-targeting strategies have now been developed to conquer the adverse consequences of ErbB2 overexpression such as paclitaxel resistance. Among these, trastuzumab has brought great promise (Yu et al., 2001). The humanized anti-p185 (HER2) monoclonal antibody trastuzumab has been shown to effectively inhibit the growth of HER2-overexpressing breast cancer cells in vivo and in vitro. The treatment of cancer cells with trastuzumab results in downregulation of the HER2 receptor. In vivo, trastuzumab induces antibody-dependent cellular cytotoxicity. Trastuzumab also inhibits constitutive HER2 cleavage/shedding mediated by metalloproteases. The ability of trastuzumab to inhibit HER2 cleavage may correlate with the clinical anticancer activity of the multifunctional HER2-targeting antibody (Baselga et al., 2001). The immunohistochemistry (IHC) performance of 4 anti-HER-2/neu antibodies was compared with fluorescent in situ hybridization (FISH) analysis of HER-2/neu gene expression in breast cancer patients considered for trastuzumab therapy (Thomson et al., 2001). The increase in the understanding of the role of growth factors and their receptors in the pathogenesis of malignancy and other undesirable hematological events taken in conjunction with the ability to produce humanized chimeric monoclonal antibodies to these targets is providing a new perspective for the treatment of leukemia, lymphoma and breast cancer, autoimmune disease and for prevention of ischemic complications. The Her2 receptor is overexpressed in select breast, ovarian, gastric and pancreatic neoplasms (Waldmann et al., 2000). Current therapeutic strategies for primary breast cancer aim to provide improvements in outcome with minimal toxicity to the patient. Thus, there is a clear need for more effective therapies. Amplification/overexpression of the human epidermal growth factor receptor-2 (HER2) is an early event in the development of a significant proportion of breast tumors. This abnormality has been shown to have a detrimental effect on prognosis, may predict the outcome of therapies such as tamoxifen and anthracyclines, and provides a target for the novel therapy, Herceptin. Herceptin is effective and well tolerated in the metastatic setting, making it an ideal candidate for use in adjuvant breast cancer therapy. This has led to the design of a number of trials that aim to provide conclusive evidence as rapidly as possible that Herceptin is well tolerated and effective in the adjuvant setting while also addressing the question of which regimen provides greatest benefit (Leyland-Jones et al., 2001). Measurement of molecular markers predictive of response to therapy should enable more selective and effective utilization of anticancer agents. In the adjuvant setting, weak, retrospective evidence suggests that tamoxifen is potentially harmful in HER2-positive patients and that there is no benefit from prolonged tamoxifen therapy. HER2 testing has become an integral part of the optimal management of the breast cancer patient (Piccart et al., 2001). Retrospective analysis revealed a higher incidence of heart failure when trastuzumab was combined with anthracyclines than that expected with anthracyclines alone. Patients experiencing cardiac dysfunction responded well to standard cardiac medication and the majority improved (Cook-Bruns et al.,

2001). Preclinical data indicate that trastuzumab has the potential for synergistic or additive effects in combination with therapies including chemotherapy and hormonal agents, providing the rationale for a number of clinical trials in women with HER2-positive metastatic breast cancer. These and other studies will identify the regimens that produce the best outcomes with the fewest possible side effects in women with HER2-positive breast cancer (Winer et al., 2001). Trastuzumab has been shown to possess significant clinical activity in metastatic breast cancer. Preclinical testing of trastuzumab combinations demonstrated additive and synergistic interactions with paclitaxel and docetaxel, respectively (Diéras et al., 2001). A similar incidence of adverse events was demonstrated in the two dose groups with the possible exception of acute infusion-related events such as fever and chills as well as rash and dyspnea, which appear to be more prevalent in the higher dose group (Vogel et al., 2001)

ACKNOWLEDGMENTS

Dorota Bartusik-Aebisher acknowledges support from the National Center of Science NCN (New drug delivery systems-MRI study, Grant OPUS-13 number 2017/25/B/ST4/02481).

REFERENCES

Aikat S, Francis GS. Trastuzumab therapy and the heart: palliation at what cost? *Congest Heart Fail.* 2001;7(4):188-190.

Albanell J, Baselga J. Unraveling resistance to trastuzumab (Herceptin): insulin-like growth factor-I receptor, a new suspect. *J Natl Cancer Inst.* 2001;93(24):1830-2.

Arteaga CL, Chinratanalab W, Carter MB. Inhibitors of HER2/neu (erbB-2) signal transduction. *Semin Oncol.* 2001;28(6 Suppl 18):30-5.

Baselga J, Albanell J, Molina MA, Arribas J. Mechanism of action of trastuzumab and scientific update. *Semin Oncol.* 2001;28(5 Suppl 16):4-11.

Bilous M; HER2 Testing Advisory Board. HER2 testing recommendations in Australia. *Pathology.* 2001; 33(4):425-7.

Cook-Bruns N. Retrospective analysis of the safety of Herceptin immunotherapy in metastatic breast cancer. *Oncology.* 2001;61 Suppl 2:58-66.

Crown J. A "bureausceptic" view of cancer drug rationing. *Lancet.* 2001;358(9294):1660.

Dank M. [Human recombinant anti-HER2 monoclonal antibody--a new targeted treatment in breast cancer]. *Orv Hetil.* 2001;142(46):2563-8.

Diéras V, Beuzeboc P, Laurence V, Pierga JY, Pouillart P. Interaction between Herceptin and taxanes. *Oncology.* 2001;61 Suppl 2:43-9.

Ensom MH, Chang TK, Patel P. Pharmacogenetics: the therapeutic drug monitoring of the future? Clin Pharmacokinet. 2001;40(11):783-802.

Fountzilas G, Tsavdaridis D, Kalogera-Fountzila A, Christodoulou CH, Timotheadou E, Kalofonos CH, Kosmidis P, Adamou A, Papakostas P, Gogas H, Stathopoulos G, Razis E, Bafaloukos D, Skarlos D. Weekly paclitaxel as first-line chemotherapy and trastuzumab in patients with advanced breast cancer. A Hellenic Cooperative Oncology Group phase II study. *Ann Oncol.* 2001;12(11):1545-51.

Freebairn AJ, Last AJ, Illidg TM. Trastuzumab: designer drug or fashionable fad? *Clin Oncol (R Coll Radiol).* 2001;13(6):427-33.

Gerber B, Krause A, Markmann S, Reimer T, Fietkau R, Müller H. Effectiveness of Trastuzumab (Herceptin) in a patient with locally recurrent breast cancer after cardiac failure caused by severe cytotoxic pretreatment. *Oncology.* 2001;61(4):271-4.

Goel S, Mani S, Perez-Soler R. Tyrosine kinase inhibitors: a clinical perspective. *Curr Oncol Rep.* 2002;4(1):9-19.

Hehl EM. Opinion on the use of the antitumor drug trastuzumab (Herceptin) in patients with metastatic breast cancer in the county Mecklenburg-Vorpommern. *Int J Clin Pharmacol Ther.* 2001;39(11):503-6.

Hortobagyi GN, Perez EA. Integration of trastuzumab into adjuvant systemic therapy of breast cancer: ongoing and planned clinical trials. *Semin Oncol.* 2001;28(5 Suppl 16):41-6. Review.

Hortobagyi GN. Optimal duration of therapy with trastuzumab. *Semin Oncol.* 2001;28(5 Suppl 16):33-40.

Hortobagyi GN. Overview of treatment results with trastuzumab (Herceptin) in metastatic breast cancer. *Semin Oncol.* 2001;28(6 Suppl 18):43-7.

Kim R, Tanabe K, Uchida Y, Osaki A, Toge T. The role of HER-2 oncoprotein in drug-sensitivity in breast cancer (review). *Oncol Rep.* 2002;9(1):3-9.

Kobayashi H, Shirakawa K, Kawamoto S, Saga T, Sato N, Hiraga A, Watanabe I, Heike Y, Togashi K, Konishi J, Brechbiel MW, Wakasugi H. Rapid accumulation and internalization of radiolabeled herceptin in an inflammatory breast cancer xenograft with vasculogenic mimicry predicted by the contrast-enhanced dynamic MRI with the macromolecular contrast agent G6-(1B4M-Gd)(256). *Cancer Res.* 2002; 62(3):860-6.

Kumar R, Yarmand-Bagheri R. The role of HER2 in angiogenesis. *Semin Oncol.* 2001;28(5 Suppl 16):27-32.

Latif Z, Watters AD, Bartlett JM, Underwood MA, Aitchison M. Gene amplification and overexpression of HER2 in renal cell carcinoma. *BJU Int.* 2002;89(1):5-9.

Leyland-Jones B, Smith I. Role of Herceptin in primary breast cancer: views from North America and Europe. *Oncology.* 2001;61 Suppl 2:83-91.

Lohrisch C, Piccart M. An overview of HER2. *Semin Oncol.* 2001;28(6 Suppl 18):3-11.

Mayfield S, Vaughn JP, Kute TE. DNA strand breaks and cell cycle perturbation in herceptin treated breast cancer cell lines. *Breast Cancer Res Treat.* 2001;70(2):123-9.

McKeage K, Perry CM. Trastuzumab: a review of its use in the treatment of metastatic breast cancer overexpressing HER2. *Drugs.* 2002;62(1):209-43.

Miles DW. Update on HER-2 as a target for cancer therapy: herceptin in the clinical setting. *Breast Cancer Res.* 2001;3(6):380-4. Epub 2001 Oct 11.

Mokbel K, Elkak A. Recent advances in breast cancer (the 37th ASCO meeting, May 2001). *Curr Med Res Opin.* 2001;17(2):116-22.

Moulder SL, Yakes FM, Muthuswamy SK, Bianco R, Simpson JF, Arteaga CL. Epidermal growth factor receptor (HER1) tyrosine kinase inhibitor ZD1839 (Iressa) inhibits HER2/neu (erbB2)-overexpressing breast cancer cells in vitro and in vivo. *Cancer Res.* 2001;61(24):8887-95.

Ohta M, Tokuda Y, Suzuki Y, Kubota M, Watanabe T, Fujii H, Sasaki Y, Niwa T, Makuuchi H, Tajima T. A case with HER2-overexpressing breast cancer completely responded to humanized anti-HER2 monoclonal antibody. *Jpn J Clin Oncol.* 2001;31(11):553-6.

Perez EA, Roche PC, Jenkins RB, Reynolds CA, Halling KC, Ingle JN, Wold LE. HER2 testing in patients with breast cancer: poor correlation between weak positivity by immunohistochemistry and gene amplification by fluorescence in situ hybridization. *Mayo Clin Proc.* 2002;77(2):148-54.

Piccart M, Lohrisch C, Di Leo A, Larsimont D. The predictive value of HER2 in breast cancer. *Oncology.* 2001;61 Suppl 2:73-82.

Piechocki MP, Pilon SA, Kelly C, Wei WZ. Degradation signals in ErbB-2 dictate proteasomal processing and immunogenicity and resist protection by cis glycine-alanine repeat. *Cell Immunol.* 2001;212(2):138-49.

Runowicz CD. Herceptin: help for advanced breast cancer. *Health News.* 2001; 7(5):4.

Savinainen KJ, Saramäki OR, Linja MJ, Bratt O, Tammela TL, Isola JJ, Visakorpi T. Expression and gene copy number analysis of ERBB2 oncogene in prostate cancer. *Am J Pathol.* 2002;160(1):339-45.

Schneider JW, Chang AY, Rocco TP. Cardiotoxicity in signal transduction therapeutics: erbB2 antibodies and the heart. *Semin Oncol.* 2001; 28(5 Suppl 16):18-26.

Sledge GW Jr. Is HER-2/neu a predictor of anthracycline utility? No. *J Natl Cancer Inst Monogr.* 2001;(30):85-7.

Slichenmyer WJ, Fry DW. Anticancer therapy targeting the erbB family of receptor tyrosine kinases. *Semin Oncol.* 2001 Oct;28(5 Suppl 16):67-79.

Sorokin P. New agents and future directions in biotherapy. *Clin J Oncol Nurs.* 2002 Jan-Feb;6(1):19-24.

Susnjar S, Bosnjak S, Radulovic S. [Trastuzumab in metastatic breast carcinoma]. *Srp Arh Celok Lek.* 2001 May-Jun;129(5-6):147-52. Review. Serbian.

Thomson TA, Hayes MM, Spinelli JJ, Hilland E, Sawrenko C, Phillips D, Dupuis B, Parker RL. HER-2/neu in breast cancer: interobserver variability and performance of immunohistochemistry with 4 antibodies compared with fluorescent in situ hybridization. *Mod Pathol.* 2001;14(11):1079-86.

Tokuda Y, Suzuki Y, Ohta M, Saito Y, Kubota M, Tajima T, Umemura S, Osamura RY. Compassionate use of humanized anti-HER2/neu protein, trastuzumab for metastatic breast cancer in Japan. *Breast Cancer.* 2001;8(4):310-5.

Umemura S, Sakamoto G, Sasano H, Tsuda H, Akiyama F, Kurosumi M, Tokuda Y, Watanabe T, Toi M, Hasegawa T, Osamura RY. Evaluation of HER2 status: for the treatment of metastatic breast cancers by humanized anti-HER2 Monoclonal antibody (trastuzumab) (Pathological committee for optimal use of trastuzumab). *Breast Cancer.* 2001;8(4):316-20. Review.

Vogel CL, Cobleigh MA, Tripathy D, Gutheil JC, Harris LN, Fehrenbacher L, Slamon DJ, Murphy M, Novotny WF, Burchmore M, Shak S, Stewart SJ, Press M. Efficacy and safety of trastuzumab as a single agent in first-line treatment of HER2-overexpressing metastatic breast cancer. *J Clin Oncol.* 2002;20(3):719-26.

Vogel CL, Cobleigh MA, Tripathy D, Gutheil JC, Harris LN, Fehrenbacher L, Slamon DJ, Murphy M, Novotny WF, Burchmore M, Shak S, Stewart SJ. First-line Herceptin monotherapy in metastatic breast cancer. *Oncology.* 2001;61 Suppl 2:37-42.

Waldmann TA, Levy R, Coller BS. Emerging Therapies: Spectrum of Applications of Monoclonal Antibody Therapy. *Hematology Am Soc Hematol Educ Program.* 2000:394-408.

Wang SC, Zhang L, Hortobagyi GN, Hung MC. Targeting HER2: recent developments and future directions for breast cancer patients. *Semin Oncol.* 2001;28(6 Suppl 18):21-9. Review.

Waterhouse DN, Tardi PG, Mayer LD, Bally MB. A comparison of liposomal formulations of doxorubicin with drug administered in free form: changing toxicity profiles. *Drug Saf.* 2001;24(12):903-20.

Winer EP, Burstein HJ. New combinations with Herceptin in metastatic breast cancer. *Oncology.* 2001;61 Suppl 2:50-7.

Wood WC. Adjuvant therapy for breast cancer: current controversies and future prospects. *J Natl Cancer Inst Monogr.* 2001;(30):16.

Yip YL, Ward RL. Anti-ErbB-2 monoclonal antibodies and ErbB-2-directed vaccines. *Cancer Immunol Immunother.* 2002;50(11):569-87.

Yu D. Mechanisms of ErbB2-mediated paclitaxel resistance and trastuzumab-mediated paclitaxel sensitization in ErbB2-overexpressing breast cancers. *Semin Oncol.* 2001;28(5 Suppl 16):12-7.

Zulkowski K, Kath R, Semrau R, Merkle K, Höffken K. Regression of brain metastases from breast carcinoma after chemotherapy with bendamustine. *J Cancer Res Clin Oncol.* 2002; 128(2):111-3.

Chapter 4

TRASTUZUMAB: PHARMACOKINETIC PROPERTIES

ABSTRACT

The pharmacokinetics of trastuzumab will be evaluated in a population pharmacokinetic model analysis using pooled data from patients with HER2 positive tumor types, and healthy volunteers. The case reports and clinical research papers will be discussed.

Keywords: trastuzmab, pharmacokinetic properties, breast cancers

INTRODUCTION

Human epidermal growth factor receptor-2 HER2 acts as a networking receptor that mediates signaling to cancer cells, causing them to proliferate. HER receptors exist as monomers but dimerize on ligand binding. HER ligands are bivalent growth factor molecules whose low-affinity site binds to HER2. HER2-containing heterodimers are relatively long-lived and potent. HER2 overexpression biases the formation of HER2-containing heterodimers, leading to enhanced responsiveness to stromal growth factors and oncogenic transformation. Removal of HER2 from the cell surface or inhibition of its intrinsic enzymatic activity may reduce oncogenicity. The reported clinical therapeutic efficacy of anti-HER2 monoclonal antibodies in breast cancer highlights the importance of understanding the biology of HER2 (Yarden et al., 2001). Trastuzumab may become future therapies for breast cancer patients (Leyland-Jones et al., 2001; Baselga et al., 2001). Although expression of the HER-2/neu oncogene has been correlated with tumor progression in prostate cancer, the biologic significance of detecting HER-2/neu gene amplification by fluorescence *in situ* hybridization or evidence for protein overexpression by immunohistochemistry remains unclear. In this study, we directly compared HER-2/neu FISH and IHC to determine which may be more predictive of the response to trastuzumab. In contrast to breast cancer, FISH detects HER-2/neu amplification in a substantial proportion of prostate cancers that do not overexpress HER-2/neuby IHC. Although the biologic significance of this finding is uncertain, it has implications for the direction of current and planned clinical trials of trastuzumab in advanced prostate cancer, including determination of patient eligibility (Liu et al., 2001). The incidence of human epidermal growth factor receptor 2 (HER2) protein overexpression and its prognostic value are not well characterized in patients with prostate cancer. A phase I study was designed to evaluate docetaxel/estramustine plus trastuzumab, a humanized monoclonal antibody that binds to the HER2 receptor, in patients with metastatic androgen-independent prostate cancer (AIPC). HER2 positivity was not required because safety was the primary endpoint.(Small et al., 2001). Taxane-induced microtubule stabilization arrests cells in the G(2)M phase of the cell cycle and induces bcl-2 phosphorylation, thereby promoting a cascade of events that ultimately leads to apoptotic cell death. In preclinical studies, docetaxel had a higher affinity for tubulin and was shown to be a more potent inducer of bcl-2 phosphorylation than paclitaxel. Laboratory evidence also supports the clinical evaluation of docetaxel-based combinations that include agents such as trastuzumab and/or estramustine. The pathways for docetaxel-induced apoptosis appear to differ in androgen-dependent and androgen-independent prostate cancer cells. Further elucidation of these differences will be instrumental in designing targeted regimens for the treatment of localized and advanced prostate cancer (Pienta et al., 2001). Anthracyclines have been in clinical practice since the 1960s and represent one of the most commonly used classes of anticancer drugs. Doxorubicin (adriamycin) is one of the first anthracyclines in clinical use, has a broad anti-tumor spectrum, and has been used against hematopoietic malignancies such as lymphoma, myeloma and leukemia, and solid tumors such as breast cancer, ovarian cancer and sarcomas. There are two chemotherapeutic regimens containing doxorubicin that have been established as the state of the art therapy against malignant lymphomas (Ogura et al., 2001; Matsumoto et al., 2001). A large body of data on systemic therapy has been presented and published in the past year, including new information on primary risk reduction, patient selection for adjuvant systemic therapy, and anthracycline-analogs. Discussions on the long-term effects of adjuvant therapy have taken center stage also. These and other important ongoing developments since 2000 are examined in this review article (Wolff et al., 2002). Most women diagnosed with primary invasive breast cancer are potential candidates to receive adjuvant systemic treatment. Tumor markers that predict the likelihood of response to therapy might help select optimal treatment for individual patients. Of these, c-erbB-2 is the most promising marker (Wolff et al., 2002; Pestalozzi et al., 2001). Overexpression of the Her-2/neu oncogene and receptor protein was reported in approximately 20% of breast cancers and was associated with a poor prognosis. Her-2/neu expression was a predictor for response to trastuzumab, a monoclonal antibody that recognizes the Her-2/neu cell surface receptor. Data regarding the expression of Her-2/neu in lung cancer are far more limited, and there is little information regarding the influence of Her-2/neu expression and response to trastuzumab alone or in combination with chemotherapeutic agents (Bunn et al., 2001). The Her2/neu (c-erbB-2) oncogene encodes a 185-kDa protein tyrosine kinase which is overexpressed in 20% of breast adenocarcinomas and is recognized by a humanized anti-Her2/neu monoclonal antibody (mAb) (rhu4D5 or Herceptin). Natural killer (NK) cells are capable of mediating antibody-dependent cell cytotoxicity (ADCC) against antibody-coated targets via their expression of a low-affinity receptor for IgG (Carson et al., 2001). Novel systemic treatments are needed in pancreatic cancer. The authors sought to establish the frequency of overexpression of the HER-2/neu oncogene in patients with pancreatic adenocarcinoma to determine the potential role of trastuzumab as a therapeutic agent in this disease. Tumor specimens from patients with pancreatic adenocarcinoma were analyzed by staining for p185HER2 protein using the DAKO immunohistochemical assay. Evaluation of the efficacy of trastuzumab for patients with pancreatic cancer who overexpress HER-2/neu appears indicated (Safran et al., 2001). The epidermal growth factor receptor (EGFR) is commonly overexpressed in many human tumors and provides a new target for anticancer drug development. ZD1839 ("Iressa"), a quinazoline tyrosine kinase inhibitor selective for the EGFR, has shown good activity in preclinical studies and in the early phase of clinical trials. However, because it remains unclear which tumor types are the best targets for treatment with this agent, the molecular characteristics that correlate with tumor sensitivity to ZD1839 have been studied. In a panel of human breast cancer and other epithelial tumor cell lines, HER2-overexpressing tumors were particularly sensitive to ZD1839 (Moasser et al., 2001). Correlation with time from initial symptoms until diagnosis, tumor size and TNM stage at diagnosis, tumor grade, type of operation and overall survival were investigated. C-erbB-2 overexpression was detected in 19.6% samples of pancreatic adenocarcinoma and in one case of Vater's ampullae carcinoma. C-erbB-2 overexpression was found in two of four insulinomas. Univariate statistical correlation stage between c-erbB-2 overexpression and time from initial symptoms until diagnosis, tumor size and TNM at diagnosis, tumor grade, type of operation and overall survival did not reach statistical significans in any parameter studied. C-erbB-2 oncogene was not found to be prognostic factor in pancreatic cancer. Its value to predict therapeutical response remains to be determined in prospective clinical trials (Moasser et al., 2001). Laboratory testing of HER2/neu in breast carcinoma has become vital to patient care following the approval of trastuzumab as the first therapy to target the HER2/neu oncoprotein. Initial clinical trials used immunohistochemistry (IHC) to test for HER2/neu overexpression in order to select patients for therapy. Fluorescence *in situ* hybridization (FISH), which tests for gene amplification, is more specific and sensitive than IHC when either assay is compared with HER2/neu overexpression as determined by Northern or Western blot analysis. Many weak overexpressors on IHC testing are not gene amplified on FISH analysis. Such weak overexpressors may be considered false-positives and raise the question of how best to test for HER2/neu. The literature was surveyed regarding testing for HER2/neu overexpression in breast carcinomas and alternative testing strategies. Most weakly positive overexpressors are false-positives on testing with FISH. Thus, screening of breast carcinomas with IHC and confirmation of weakly positive IHC results by FISH is an effective evolving strategy for testing HER2/neu as a predictor of response to targeted therapy (Diaz et al., 2001; Zulkowski et al., 2002), (Leslie et al., 2002; Runowicz et al., 2001; Hehl et al., 2001; Gerber et al., 2001;Slichenmyer et al., 2001;Hortobagyi et al., 2001;Hortobagyi et al., 2001; Kumar et al., 2001; Schneider et al., 2001; Yu et al., 2001; Baselga et al., 2001; Thomson et al., 2001; Waldmann et al., 2000; Leyland-Jones et al., 2001; Piccart et al., 2001; Cook-Bruns et al., 2001; Rudlowski et al., 2001, Strasser et al., 2001, Strasser et al., 2001, Behr et al., 2001). Salivary duct carcinoma (SDC) is a highly malignant salivary gland tumor with aggressive clinical behavior, and is characterized by its histological resemblance to invasive ductal carcinoma of the breast. Overexpression and/or amplification of proto-oncogene Her2/neu has been shown to influence both prognosis and treatment of breast cancer. Since salivary duct carcinoma and ductal breast carcinoma share many common characteristics, HER2/neu overexpression might also be important in SDC (Skálová et al., 2001). Evaluation of HER-2/neu status is important in the management of patients with breast carcinoma, especially in determining the possible application of trastuzumab, a humanized anti-HER-2/neu monoclonal antibody. Chromogenic *in situ* hybridization (CISH) detection of the HER-2/neu oncogene is a newly developed *in situ* hybridization method that utilizes a robust and unique-sequence DNA probe labeled with digoxygenin, and sequential incubations with antidigoxygenin fluorescein, antifluorescein peroxidase, and diaminobenzidine. Gene copy signals for

HER-2/neu were recognized as intranuclear brown dots in both neoplastic and non-neoplastic cells. Seven carcinomas showed an increased number or size of signals and were interpreted as being positive for HER-2/neu amplification. Eight cases were positive with the HercepTest. Seven out of eight carcinoma cases found to overexpress immunoreactive HER-2/neu also demonstrated HER-2/neu gene amplification following CISH analysis (Kumamoto et al., 2001). Breast cancer is the most common malignancy in women in the United States in the year 2000. The proto-oncogene Her-2/neu (c-erb-B2) has become an increasingly important prognostic and predictive factor in breast cancer. Overexpression/amplification of the Her-2/neu has been associated with a worse outcome in patients with breast cancer. Herceptin, a "humanized" murine monoclonal antibody directed against the extracellular domain of the Her-2/neu protein, is being used to treat breast cancer that overexpresses Her-2/neu. The status of Her-2/neu in the tumor has become a critical factor in the management strategy of a breast cancer patient. The objective of this article is to provide a comprehensive review of all aspects of Her-2/neu in breast cancer, including biology, prognostic and predictive value, targeted Herceptin therapy, and the laboratory testing of Her-2/neu (Kaptain et al., 2001). Breast cancer research has developed at a rapid pace over the last decades. Recent discoveries promise to provide individualized treatment options, increased long-term survival for women with breast cancer, and the possibility of moving toward curative intent in the treatment of advanced breast cancer. Age, race, tumor size, histological tumor type, axillary nodal status, standardized pathological grade, and hormone-receptor status are accepted as established prognostic and/or predictive factors for selection of systemic adjuvant treatment of breast cancer. The role of other promising new factors, such as p53 mutations, HER-2 status, plasminogen activator system, histological evidence of vascular invasion, and quantitative parameters of angiogenesis will be determined in ongoing prospective studies. Currently, 5 years' treatment with adjuvant tamoxifen in women with hormone-positive receptor status, is regarded as the optimal duration of treatment. Long-term follow-up on the randomized trials will determine the added benefit of treatment beyond 5 years. Ovarian ablation has shown a reduction in recurrence and death, and the exact role and extent of adjuvant chemotherapy in premenopausal women with hormone-responsive tumors is under discussion. Combination hormonal and chemo-hormonal therapies are also being evaluated. There are no convincing data on the survival impact of tamoxifen as a preventative therapy for breast cancer: longer-term follow-up is required, and the planned meta-analyses in 2005 should help shed light on this issue. Statistically significant benefits have been observed with adjuvant chemotherapy (particularly with anthracycline-containing regimens in premenopausal women) versus no adjuvant chemotherapy (Aapro et al., 2001, (Livingston et al., 2001; Field et al., 2001). The arrival of Herceptin (Trastuzumab), an antibody against the HER2 oncogene found in a proportion of breast carcinomas and other carcinomas, has emphasised the need for a standardised technique for demonstrating overexpression of HER2 (Field et al., 2001; Schaller et al., 2001). A significant number of women with advanced breast cancer fail to respond to standard-dose chemotherapy. Trastuzumab as monotherapy or in combination with paclitaxel or other non-anthracyclines (Mrsić et al., 2001). The HER family of receptors has an important role in the network of cell signals controlling cell growth and differentiation. Although the activity of the HER receptor is strictly controlled in normal cells, HER2 receptor overexpression plays a pivotal role in transformation and tumorigenesis. HER2 gene overexpression of the receptor has been detected in subsets of a wide range of human cancers including breast cancer, and is an indicator of poor prognosis. It is proposed that overexpressed HER2 causes high activity of cell-signaling networks, thereby resulting in tumor cell proliferation. HER2 receptor is an attractive target for new anti-cancer treatments. The anti-tumor mechanisms of anti-HER2 monoclonal antibodies are not completely understood. However, some tumor types are not sensitive to trastuzumab, suggesting that the response of a tumor to trastuzumab may not only be dependent on overexpressed HER2, but may also be influenced by other members of the HER receptor family expressed in the tumor cel 1 (Neve et al., 2001). HER2 is overexpressed/amplified in 20%-30% of human breast tumors and is a marker for a poor prognosis. For these reasons, HER2 has been selected as a therapeutic target for breast cancer treatment. Oncologists can no longer ignore the importance of HER2 status for treatment algorithms in breast cancer (Piccart et al., 2001; Smith et al., 2001; Bell et al., 2001). One of the major expectations from the use of humanized monoclonal antibodies in cancer therapy has been that of exploiting the specificity and sensitivity of the immune system to achieve selective therapeutic effects devoid of the often severe toxicity caused by chemotherapy. The incidence of severe or serious adverse effects attributable to trastuzumab was low (Gianni et al., 2001; Eiermann et al., 2001; Baselga et al., 2001). Trastuzumab when administered on a weekly schedule either alone or in combination with taxanes, improves survival of women with HER2-positive metastatic breast cancer (Leyland-Jones et al., 2001). The search for new methods of treating cancer, combined with advances in our understanding of carcinogenesis, molecular biology and technology, has resulted in the development of novel biologic agents with proven clinical efficacy. One such agent is trastuzumab (Herceptin), a humanized monoclonal antibody that targets the human epidermal growth factor receptor-2. HER2 is a member of a family of receptors that interact with each other and various ligands to stimulate various intracellular signal transduction pathways involved in cell growth control. This paper reviews current knowledge of the mechanism of action of trastuzumab, including. The significance of these mechanisms for selection of concomitant chemotherapy is also considered (Baselga et al., 2001). A range of growth factors serve as ligands, but none is specific for the HER2 receptor. Ligand binding to HERI, HER3 or HER4 induces rapid receptor dimerization, with a marked preference for HER2 as a dimer partner. When HER2 is overexpressed multiple HER2 heterodimers are formed and cell signaling is stronger, resulting in enhanced responsiveness to growth factors and malignant growth. This explains why HER2 overexpression is an indicator of poor prognosis in breast tumors and may be predictive of response to treatment. HER2 is a highly specific and promising target for new breast cancer treatments (Rubin et al., 2001). In recent years investigators have looked at the human epidermal growth factor receptor-2 (HER2), which is overexpressed in 20%-30% of breast cancer patients, with regard to its role as a prognostic and predictive factor. Although many studies have suggested that HER2 overexpression may be associated with a poor clinical outcome, other studies have not fully supported this observation. The inconsistencies between studies may be due in part to discrepancies between different HER2 testing methods. The application of this method demonstrated that 85% of all breast tumor samples expressed HER2 at levels greater than normal. The investigation of HER2 status as a predictor of response to therapy has also yielded many conflicting results. With the development of targeted anti-HER2 therapies, assessment of HER2 status will be important in stratifying patients to the most appropriate treatment regimens (Cooke et al., 2001; Lane et al., 2001). To date, poor standardization in HER2 status evaluation has precluded reliable comparison of overexpression rates in different tumors. However, standardized methodologies have been introduced recently for these analyses, and have identified frequencies of 51%, 44%, 26% and 25% in Wilm's tumor, bladder, pancreatic and breast carcinoma, respectively. Other tumors tested had frequencies below 20%. The frequency was greater than that predicted by gene amplification data in some tumor types, which may indicate overexpression due to gene deregulation, rather than gene amplification. Analysis of a large retrospective series of breast carcinomas demonstrated an association between HER2 positivity and a number of other prognostic markers (Ménard et al., 2001). Low-molecular-weight inhibitors of the EGFR tyrosine kinase also in clinical development include OSI-774, PD182905, PKI-166, CI-1033, and ZD1839. ZD1839 has shown encouraging results in patients with prostate cancer in phase 1 trials (Barton et al., 2001). The idea of using the specificity of antibodies to target malignant cells was put forward very soon after the discovery of techniques to generate monoclonal reagents. The responses seen with mouse anti-idiotype in patients with B-cell lymphomas indicated the potential of this approach, but it was some years before key technical obstacles were overcome and the more widespread application of these therapies became possible. Whilst they were originally conceived as having an immunotherapeutic effect, it has become clear that recruitment of immune effectors is only one component of successful antibody therapy, and their action upon the cellular target, either blocking or agonistic, is also critical. The development of immunoconjugates to deliver toxins or radiation is a further extension of the approach, and here again the intracellular effect of antibody ligation appears to be crucial. This presentation will address the central theme of antibody treatments for malignancy that are now reaching the clinic, and will use these examples to highlight ways in which antibodies may be acting *in vivo* (Johnson et al., 2001). Adjuvant chemotherapy in breast cancer has clearly been shown to reduce mortality. The benefits extend to pre- and postmenopausal women and those with node-negative, node-positive, estrogen receptor (ER)-positive, and ER-negative disease. Updated data regarding chemoendocrine therapy in postmenopausal women and anthracycline-based regimens are presented. Dose intensity, dose density, and high-dose therapy have not been proven efficacious to date, but further trials are pending. The incorporation of taxanes and bisphosphonates has been further elucidated, with follow-up studies in progress. The potential role of trastuzumab is the focus of several clinical trials. Recent findings regarding the long-term side effects of adjuvant therapy are reviewed (Tan et al., 2001). Cytotoxic chemotherapy is important for treatment of women with hormone-insensitive or hormone-refractory advanced breast cancer. A variety of agents are effective, alone or in combination. The clinical activity and side effects of many agents, as well as principles for use of chemotherapy, are reviewed. The growing availability of such biological therapies given in combination with chemotherapy may mean better survival in the future for women with advanced breast cancer (Burstein et al., 2001). Recent studies suggest that HER-2/neu specifically promotes the invasive capacity of tumor cells by up-regulating secretion of the proteolytic enzyme, urokinase-type plasminogen activator (uPA), or its inhibitor, plasminogen activator inhibitor-1 (PAI-1), in colon and gastric cancer (Konecny et al., 2001). Furthermore, a full-length human HER-2/neu cDNA was introduced into five human breast cancer cell lines to define the effects of HER-2/neu overexpression on uPA and PAI-1 expression. The present findings suggest that the invasive phenotype elicited by HER-2/neu overexpression in breast cancer is not a direct effect of uPA or PAI-1 expression. HER-2/neu and the uPA/PAI-1 axis have been shown to affect the invasive capacity of breast cancer independently (Konecny et al., 2001). Immunoliposomes were constructed using a modular strategy in which components were optimized for internalization and intracellular drug delivery. Repeat administrations revealed no increase in clearance, further confirming that ILs retain the long circulation and non-immunogenicity of sterically stabilized liposomes. In five different HER2-overexpressing xenograft models, anti-HER2 ILs loaded with doxorubicin (dox) showed potent anticancer activity, including tumor inhibition, regressions, and cures (pathologic complete responses). In a non-HER2-overexpressing xenograft model (MCF7), ILs and non-targeted liposomal dox produced equivalent antitumor effects. Detailed studies of tumor localization indicated a novel mechanism of drug delivery for anti-HER2 ILs. However, histologic studies using colloidal-gold labeled ILs demonstrated efficient intracellular delivery in tumor cells, while non-targeted liposomes accumulated within stroma, either extracellularly or within macrophages. Finally, further studies of the mechanism of action of anti-HER2 ILs-dox suggest that this strategy may provide optimal delivery of anthracycline-based chemotherapy to HER2-overexpressing cancer cells in the clinic, while circumventing the cardiotoxicity associated with trastuzumab + anthracycline (Park et al., 2001). Despite progressive developments in therapeutic interventions, including surgery, radiotherapy and chemotherapy, there has been no major improvement in the survival of women with metastatic breast cancer (MBC). Based on knowledge of tumor growth patterns, approaches addressing this issue have included increasing chemotherapy dose or dose density and extending the duration of therapy. However, only the latter approach has resulted in improved clinical benefit, although not survival; and its use is restricted by the cumulative toxicity of chemotherapeutic agents. The preclinical and clinical findings on which the current recommended duration of Herceptin therapy are based are reviewed and alternative strategies are discussed (Bell et al., 2001). Only 25% of patients with HER-2/neu-positive metastatic breast tumors respond favorably to trastuzamab (Herceptin) treatment. (Simon et al., 2001). HER-2/neu (ERB-B2), a member of the receptor tyrosine kinase superfamily, is altered by gene amplification and/or protein overexpression in a wide variety of human epithelial malignancies. Such alterations activate signaling systems that promote cell growth, angiogenesis, cancer metastases, and other procarcinogenic pathways (1). These HER-2 abnormalities are found in approximately one third of breast cancers. HER-2 "status" is a loose and suboptimal term that is commonly used to describe the degree of HER-2 gene amplification and/or the extent of Her-2 protein overexpression. Statistically significant interactions between HER-2 status and chemotherapeutic agents other than anthracyclines have also been reported. Given these chemotherapeutic/HER-2 interactions and new anti-HER-2 therapeutic agents, it is no longer always correct to assume that cancers with an altered HER-2 status will have a poor outcome. As noted, HER-2 has become an important target for novel therapeutic strategies, such as trastuzumab (Herceptin), a monoclonal antibody that acts as an HER-2 antagonist. This agent has shown promise in treating a subset of patients with otherwise chemorefractory, late-stage breast cancer. Many recently opened breast cancer trials combine Herceptin with other agents to treat various stages of disease (Thor et al., 2001). HER2 overexpression occurs in 25% of breast cancers and seems to correlate with poor prognosis. HER2 overexpression may predict tamoxifen failure and different response rates to chemotherapeutic agents such as the taxanes and anthracyclines. Currently, Trastuzumab and paclitaxel is the only combination indicated for the treatment of patients with metastatic breast cancer whose tumours overexpress HER2. It is also indicated as a single agent in women with HER2-overexpressing metastatic breast cancer that has progressed after previous chemotherapy. Herceptin is a well-tolerated drug and the side-effects that are commonly seen with chemotherapy, such as neutropenia, alopecia and mucositis, are rarely observed. The main risk factors for cardiotoxicity are concurrent or previous anthracycline exposure (Thor et al., 2001). HER2 therapy of human HER2/neu expressing malignancies such as breast cancer has shown only partial success in clinical trials. In addition to antibodies, compounds that directly inhibit receptor tyrosine kinases have shown preclinical activity and early clinical activity has been reported (Mendelsohn et al., 2000; Mokbel et al., 2001; Lu et al., 2001;Albanell et al., 2001;Moulder et al., 2001; Piechocki et al., 2001;Kim et al., 2002;Miles et al., 2001; Waterhouse et al., 2001; Ensom et al., 2001;Goel et al., 2001;Crown et al., 2001). Moreover, it is an entry criterion in the assessment of patients for whom Trastuzumab treatment is considered. The overexpression rate of HER2 oncoprotein has been identified in 10% to 40% of human breast cancers. In Taiwan, a higher grade of pathobiologic characteristics of familial breast cancer was also noted than that found in the non-familial group. The overexpression rate is higher in the familial breast cancer group when compared with non-familial breast cancer group, which did not prove to be statistically significant. However, when the infiltrating ductal carcinomas of both groups are compared, it is statistically significant. Overexpression correlated with node status and histological grade of infiltrating ductal carcinomas in non-familial and overall breast cancers. It also correlated with nuclear pleomorphism and mitotic counts, but not tubule formation or tumor size. All 3 cases of Paget's disease revealed overexpression, whereas all 12 cases of mucinous and one case of metaplastic carcinoma and one case of medullary carcinoma were negative. This suggests that overexpression decreases within individual tumors as they evolve from *in situ* to invasive lesioins. Although the overexpression rate of HER-2/neu oncoprotein of familial breast cancer was not significantly higher than that of the non-familial group, it is appropriate to evaluate the rate of HER-2/neu overexpression according to the histological type of breast cancers from familial breast cancer and non-familial breast cancer (Tsai et al., 2001). The combination resulted in an enhancement of TRAIL-mediated apoptosis in all cell lines overexpressing erbB-2 receptor compared with either reagent alone. In contrast, there was no effect in cell lines with low levels of the erb-B2 receptor. Trastuzumab treatment resulted in down-regulation of the erbB-2 receptor in all erbB-2-overexpressing cell lines. Similar enhancement of TRAIL toxicity was observed when the erbB-2 receptor was down-regulated using antisense oligodeoxynucleotides. Expression of a constitutively active form of Akt kinase in an erbB-2-overexpressing cell line completely abrogated the increase in TRAIL-mediated apoptosis by trastuzumab and significantly reduced the biological effect of either reagent alone. Therefore, down-regulation of the erbB-2 receptor by trastuzumab enhances TRAIL-mediated apoptosis by inhibiting Akt kinase activity. These data suggest that the combination of trastuzumab and TRAIL may allow enhanced therapeutic efficacy and specificity in the treatment of erbB-2-overexpressing tumors (Cuello et al., 2001). This inhibitory effect of trastuzumab was not shared by 2C4, an antibody against a different epitope of the HER2 ectodomain. The inhibition of basal and APMA-induced cleavage of HER2 by trastuzumab preceded antibody-induced receptor down-modulation, which indicated that the effect of trastuzumab on cleavage was not attributable to a decrease in cell-surface HER2 induced by trastuzumab. (Molina et al., 2001; Meden et al., 2001; McKeage et al., 2002; Savinainen et al., 2002; Hortobagyi et al., 2001; Arteaga et al., 2001;Wang et al., 2001; Lohrisch et al., 2001;Sledge et al., 2001;Wood et al., 2001;Ohta et al., 2001;Dank et al., 2001;Mayfield et al., 2001;Mueller-Holzner et al., 2001). Breast cancer is the most frequent type of cancer in women. The therapeutic approaches to breast cancer have developed rapidly over the past 20 years, due to the increasing knowledge about the biology of breast cancer. Therefore it was possible to increase response rates as well as the duration of response and survival in neoadjuvant, adjuvant, and palliative treatment. This paper gives a review of the current breast cancer trials. Effective new cytotoxic chemotherapy and hormonal therapy agents, as well as the identification of specific molecular abnormalities (HER2/neu) led to the development of targeted therapeutic interventions in the neoadjuvant, adjuvant, and palliative treatment of breast cancer. Increased understanding of the biology of breast cancer led to the development of rational therapeutic interventions, which are currently under active clinical development (Wenzel et al., 2001; Barthélémy et al., 2014; Huynh et al., 2014; Hayashi et al., 2015; Li et al., 2014; Li et al., 2014; Andjelić-Dekić et al., 2014; Miolo et al., 2014; Li et al., 2014; Cinar et al., 2014; Di Lisi et al., 2016; Latif et al., 2002; Sorokin et al., 2002; Perez et al., 2002; Kobayashi et al., 2002; Aikat et al., 2001; Bilous, 2001; Fountzilas et al., 2001; Vogel et al., 200; Yip et al., 2002; Susnjar et al., 2001; Umemura et al., 2001; Tokuda et al., 2001). Breast cancer is the most common cancer among women in the United States. The administration of certain types of chemotherapy may put breast cancer survivors at risk for late effect drug-induced congestive heart failure (CHF). This case study discusses the diagnosis, management, and follow-up of drug-induced CHF in a woman with breast cancer. (Moore et al., 2001). The cyclooxygenase 2 (COX-2) and ErbB/HER pathways are important modulators of cancer cell growth. A cell-proliferation assay was used to determine the response of HCA-7 cells to the HER-3/HER-4 ligand heregulin beta-1 (HRGbeta-1 Therefore, targeting of both the COX-2 and ErbB signaling pathways may represent a novel approach for the treatment and/or prevention of colorectal cancer in humans Mann et al., 2001(Gillham et al., 2001 v (Ficorella et al., 2001; Winer et al., 2001;Diéras et al., 2001;Vogel et al., 2001; Pivot et al., 2015;Foekens et al., 2015;Marano et al., 2015; Advani et al., 2015; Selcukbiricik et al., 2015; Jordan et al., 2015; Yu et al., 2015; Pircher et al., 2015; Karagöz et al., 2015; Skopets et al., 2015; Xue et al., 2014; Jitawatanarat et al., 2014; Bousquet et al., 2016; Dang et al., 2015; Tansi et al., 2015; Elster et al., 2015; Sueta et al., 2014; Thill et al., 2015; Thill et al., 2015; Pierga et al., 2015; Jakovljevic et al., 2014; Kocar et al., 2014). To determine the response rate and toxicity profile of trastuzumab administered concurrently with weekly vinorelbine in women with HER2-overexpressing advanced breast cancer. Forty women with HER2-positive (+3 by immunohistochemistry, n = 30; +2 or positive, n = 10) breast cancer thereafter) and vinorelbine (25 mg/m2 weekly, with dose adjusted each week for neutrophil count). Combination therapy was feasible; patients received concurrent trastuzumab and vinorelbine in 93% of treatment weeks. Neutropenia was the only grade 4 toxicity. No patients had symptomatic heart failure. Grade 2 cardiac toxicity was observed in three patients. Prior cumulative doxorubicin dose in excess of 240 mg/m2 and borderline pre-existing cardiac function were associated with grade 2 cardiac toxicity (Galligioni et al., 2001, Burstein et al., 2001).

ACKNOWLEDGMENTS

Dorota Bartusik-Aebisher acknowledges support from the National Center of Science NCN (New drug delivery systems-MRI study, Grant OPUS-13 number 2017/25/B/ST4/02481).

REFERENCES

Aapro, MS. Adjuvant therapy of primary breast cancer: a review of key findings from the 7th international conference, St. Gallen, February 2001. *Oncologist.*, 2001, 6(4), 376-85.

Advani, PP; Crozier, JA; Perez, EA. HER2 testing and its predictive utility in anti-HER2 breast cancer therapy. *Biomark Med.*, 2015, 9(1), 35-49.

Advani, PP; Crozier, JA; Perez, EA. HER2 testing and its predictive utility in anti-HER2 breast cancer therapy. *Biomark Med.*, 2015, 9(1), 35-49.

Aikat, S; Francis, GS. Trastuzumab therapy and the heart: palliation at what cost? *Congest Heart Fail.*, 2001, 7(4), 188-190.

Aikat, S; Francis, GS. Trastuzumab therapy and the heart: palliation at what cost? *Congest Heart Fail.*, 2001, 7(4), 188-190.

Albanell, J; Baselga, J. Unraveling resistance to trastuzumab (Herceptin): insulin-like growth factor-I receptor, a new suspect. *J Natl Cancer Inst.*, 2001, 93(24), 1830-2. No abstract available.

Albanell, J; Baselga, J. Unraveling resistance to trastuzumab (Herceptin): insulin-like growth factor-I receptor, a new suspect. *J Natl Cancer Inst.*, 2001, 93(24), 1830-2. No abstract available.

Andjelić-Dekić, N; Božović-Spasojević, I; Milošević, S; Matijašević, M; Karadžić, K. A rare case of isolated adrenal metastasis of invasive ductal breast carcinoma. *Srp Arh Celok Lek.*, 2014, 142(9-10), 597-601.

Andjelić-Dekić, N; Božović-Spasojević, I; Milošević, S; Matijašević, M; Karadžić, K. A rare case of isolated adrenal metastasis of invasive ductal breast carcinoma. *Srp Arh Celok Lek.*, 2014, 142(9-10), 597-601.

Arteaga, CL; Chinratanalab, W; Carter, MB. Inhibitors of HER2/neu (erbB-2) signal transduction. *Semin Oncol.*, 2001, 28(6 Suppl 18), 30-5.

Arteaga, CL; Chinratanalab, W; Carter, MB. Inhibitors of HER2/neu (erbB-2) signal transduction. *Semin Oncol.*, 2001, 28, (6 Suppl 18), 30-5.

Baculi, RH; Suki, S; Nisbett, J; Leeds, N; Groves, M. Meningeal carcinomatosis from breast carcinoma responsive to trastuzumab. *J Clin Oncol.*, 2001, 19(13), 3297-8.

Barbareschi, M; Doglioni, C. [Herceptin: a new drug finding new life in the determination of c-erb-B2 in breast cancer]. *Pathologica.*, 2001 93(2), 139-40. Italian.

Barthélémy, P; Leblanc, J; Wendling, F; Wissler, MP; Bergerat, JP. [Pertuzumab and solid tumors: perspectives]. *Bull Cancer.*, 2014, 101(12), 1114-21.

Barton, J; Blackledge, G; Wakeling, A. Growth factors and their receptors: new targets for prostate cancer therapy. *Urology.*, 2001, 58, (2 Suppl 1), 114-22.

Baselga, J; Albanell, J; Molina, MA; Arribas, J. Mechanism of action of trastuzumab and scientific update. *Semin Oncol.*, 2001, 28, (5 Suppl 16), 4-11.

Baselga, J; Albanell, J. Mechanism of action of anti-HER2 monoclonal antibodies. *Ann Oncol.*, 2001, 12 Suppl 1, S35-41.

Baselga, J. Herceptin alone or in combination with chemotherapy in the treatment of HER2-positive metastatic breast cancer: pivotal trials. *Oncology.*, 2001, 61, Suppl 2, 14-21.

Baselga, J. Phase I and II clinical trials of trastuzumab. *Ann Oncol.*, 2001, 12, Suppl 1, S49-55.

Behr, TM; Béhé, M; Wörmann, B. Trastuzumab and breast cancer. *N Engl J Med.*, 2001, 345(13), 995-6.

Bell, R. Duration of therapy in metastatic breast cancer: management using Herceptin. *Anticancer Drugs.*, 2001, 12(7), 561-8.

Bell, R. Ongoing trials with trastuzumab in metastatic breast cancer. *Ann Oncol.*, 2001, 12 Suppl, 1, S69-73.

Bilous, M. HER2 Testing Advisory Board. HER2 testing recommendations in Australia. *Pathology.*, 2001, 33(4), 425-7.

Bilous, M. HER2 Testing Advisory Board. HER2 testing recommendations in Australia. *Pathology.*, 2001, 33(4), 425-7. Review.

Bousquet, G; Darrouzain, F; de Bazelaire, C; Ternant, D; Barranger, E; Winterman, S; Madelaine-Chambin, I; Thiebaut, JB; Polivka, M; Paintaud, G; Culine, S; Janin, A. Intrathecal Trastuzumab Halts Progression of CNS Metastases in Breast Cancer. *J Clin Oncol.*, 2016, 34(16), e151-5.

Bousquet, G; Darrouzain, F; de Bazelaire, C; Ternant, D; Barranger, E; Winterman, S; Madelaine-Chambin, I; Thiebaut, JB; Polivka, M; Paintaud, G; Culine, S; Janin, A. Intrathecal Trastuzumab Halts Progression of CNS Metastases in Breast Cancer. *J Clin Oncol.*, 2016, 34(16), e151-5.

Bunn, PA; Jr. Helfrich, B; Soriano, AF; Franklin, WA; Varella-Garcia, M; Hirsch, FR; Baron, A; Zeng, C; Chan, DC. Expression of Her-2/neu in human lung cancer cell lines by immunohistochemistry and fluorescence *in situ* hybridization and its relationship to *in vitro* cytotoxicity by trastuzumab and chemotherapeutic agents. *Clin Cancer Res.*, 2001, 7(10), 3239-50.

Burstein, HJ; Bunnell, CA; Winer, EP. New cytotoxic agents and schedules for advanced breast cancer. *Semin Oncol.*, 2001, 28(4), 344-58.

Burstein, HJ; Kuter, I; Campos, SM; Gelman, RS; Tribou, L; Parker, LM; Manola, J; Younger, J; Matulonis, U; Bunnell, CA; Partridge, AH; Richardson, PG; Clarke, K; Shulman, LN; Winer, EP. Clinical activity of trastuzumab and vinorelbine in women with HER2-overexpressing metastatic breast cancer. *J Clin Oncol.*, 2001, 19(10), 2722-30.

Carson, WE; Parihar, R; Lindemann, MJ; Personeni, N; Dierksheide, J; Meropol, NJ; Baselga, J; Caligiuri, MA. Interleukin-2 enhances the natural killer cell response to Herceptin-coated Her2/neu-positive breast cancer cells. *Eur J Immunol.*, 2001, 31(10), 3016-25.

Cinar, P; Calkins, SM; Venook, AP; Kelley, RK. A case series of patients with HER2-overexpressed primary metastatic gastroesophageal adenocarcinoma. *Anticancer Res.*, 2014, 34(12), 7357-60.

Cinar, P; Calkins, SM; Venook, AP; Kelley, RK. A case series of patients with HER2-overexpressed primary metastatic gastroesophageal adenocarcinoma. *Anticancer Res.*, 2014, 34(12), 7357-60.

Cook-Bruns, N. Retrospective analysis of the safety of Herceptin immunotherapy in metastatic breast cancer. *Oncology.*, 2001, 61, Suppl 2, 58-66.

Cook-Bruns, N. Retrospective analysis of the safety of Herceptin immunotherapy in metastatic breast cancer. *Oncology.*, 2001, 61, Suppl 2, 58-66.

Cooke, T; Reeves, J; Lanigan, A; Stanton, P. HER2 as a prognostic and predictive marker for breast cancer. *Ann Oncol.*, 2001, 12, Suppl 1, S23-8.

Crown, J. A "bureausceptic" view of cancer drug rationing. *Lancet.*, 2001, 358(9294), 1660.

Crown, J. A "bureausceptic" view of cancer drug rationing. *Lancet.*, 2001, 358(9294), 1660.

Cuello, M; Ettenberg, SA; Clark, AS; Keane, MM; Posner, RH; Nau, MM; Dennis, PA; Lipkowitz, S. Down-regulation of the erbB-2 receptor by trastuzumab (herceptin) enhances tumor necrosis factor-related apoptosis-inducing ligand-mediated apoptosis in breast and ovarian cancer cell lines that overexpress erbB-2. *Cancer Res.*, 2001, 61(12), 4892-900.

Dang, C; Iyengar, N; Datko, F; D'Andrea, G; Theodoulou, M; Dickler, M; Goldfarb, S; Lake, D; Fasano, J; Fornier, M; Gilewski, T; Modi, S; Gajria, D; Moynahan, ME; Hamilton, N; Patil, S; Jochelson, M; Norton, L; Baselga, J; Hudis, C. Phase II study of paclitaxel given once per week along with trastuzumab and pertuzumab in patients with human epidermal growth factor receptor 2-positive metastatic breast cancer. *J Clin Oncol.*, 2015, 33(5), 442-7.

Dang, C; Iyengar, N; Datko, F; D'Andrea, G; Theodoulou, M; Dickler, M; Goldfarb, S; Lake, D; Fasano, J; Fornier, M; Gilewski, T; Modi, S;

Gajria, D; Moynahan, ME; Hamilton, N; Patil, S; Jochelson, M; Norton, L; Baselga, J; Hudis, C. Phase II study of paclitaxel given once per week along with trastuzumab and pertuzumab in patients with human epidermal growth factor receptor 2-positive metastatic breast cancer. *J Clin Oncol.*, 2015, 33(5), 442-7.

Dank, M. [Human recombinant anti-HER2 monoclonal antibody--a new targeted treatment in breast cancer]. *Orv Hetil.*, 2001, 142(46), 2563-8.

Dank, M. [Human recombinant anti-HER2 monoclonal antibody--a new targeted treatment in breast cancer]. *Orv Hetil.*, 2001, 142(46), 2563-8.

Di Lisi, D; Leggio, G; Vitale, G; Arrotti, S; Iacona, R; Inciardi, RM; Nobile, D; Bonura, F; Novo, G; Russo, A; Novo, S. Chemotherapy cardiotoxicity: cardioprotective drugs and early identification of cardiac dysfunction. *J Cardiovasc Med* (Hagerstown)., 2016, 17(4), 270-5.

Di Lisi, D; Leggio, G; Vitale, G; Arrotti, S; Iacona, R; Inciardi, RM; Nobile, D; Bonura, F; Novo, G; Russo, A; Novo, S. Chemotherapy cardiotoxicity: cardioprotective drugs and early identification of cardiac dysfunction. *J Cardiovasc Med* (Hagerstown)., 2016, 17(4), 270-5.

Diaz, NM. Laboratory testing for HER2/neu in breast carcinoma: an evolving strategy to predict response to targeted therapy. *Cancer Control.*, 2001, 8(5), 415-8.

Diéras, V; Beuzeboc, P; Laurence, V; Pierga, JY; Pouillart, P. Interaction between Herceptin and taxanes. *Oncology.*, 2001, 61, Suppl 2, 43-9.

Diéras, V; Beuzeboc, P; Laurence, V; Pierga, JY; Pouillart, P. Interaction between Herceptin and taxanes. *Oncology.*, 2001, 61, Suppl 2, 43-9.

Eiermann, W. International Herceptin Study Group. Trastuzumab combined with chemotherapy for the treatment of HER2-positive metastatic breast cancer: pivotal trial data. *Ann Oncol.*, 2001, 12, Suppl 1, S57-62.

Elster, N; Collins, DM; Toomey, S; Crown, J; Eustace, AJ; Hennessy, BT. HER2-family signalling mechanisms, clinical implications and targeting in breast cancer. *Breast Cancer Res Treat.*, 2015, 149(1), 5-15.

Elster, N; Collins, DM; Toomey, S; Crown, J; Eustace, AJ; Hennessy, BT. HER2-family signalling mechanisms, clinical implications and targeting in breast cancer. *Breast Cancer Res Treat.*, 2015, 149(1), 5-15.

Ensom, MH; Chang, TK; Patel, P. Pharmacogenetics: the therapeutic drug monitoring of the future? *Clin Pharmacokinet.*, 2001, 40(11), 783-802.

Ensom, MH; Chang, TK; Patel, P. Pharmacogenetics: the therapeutic drug monitoring of the future? *Clin Pharmacokinet.*, 2001, 40(11), 783-802.

Ficorella, C. [Docetaxel (Taxotere) in combination with trastuzumab (Herceptin)]. *Tumori.*, 2001, 87, (1 Suppl 2), S10-8.

Field, AS; Chamberlain, NL; Tran, D; Morey, AL. Suggestions for HER-2/neu testing in breast carcinoma, based on a comparison of immunohistochemistry and fluorescence *in situ* hybridisation. *Pathology.*, 2001, 33(3), 278-82.

Foekens, JA; Martens, JW; Sleijfer, S. Are immune signatures a worthwhile tool for decision making in early-stage human epidermal growth factor receptor 2-positive breast cancer? *J Clin Oncol.*, 2015, 33(7), 673-5.

Foekens, JA; Martens, JW; Sleijfer, S. Are immune signatures a worthwhile tool for decision making in early-stage human epidermal growth factor receptor 2-positive breast cancer? *J Clin Oncol.*, 2015, 33(7), 673-5.

Fountzilas, G; Tsavdaridis, D; Kalogera-Fountzila, A; Christodoulou, CH; Timotheadou, E; Kalofonos, CH; Kosmidis, P; Adamou, A; Papakostas, P; Gogas, H; Stathopoulos, G; Razis, E; Bafaloukos, D; Skarlos, D. Weekly paclitaxel as first-line chemotherapy and trastuzumab in patients with advanced breast cancer. A Hellenic Cooperative Oncology Group phase II study. *Ann Oncol.*, 2001, 12(11), 1545-51.

Fountzilas, G; Tsavdaridis, D; Kalogera-Fountzila, A; Christodoulou, CH; Timotheadou, E; Kalofonos, CH; Kosmidis, P; Adamou, A; Papakostas, P; Gogas, H; Stathopoulos, G; Razis, E; Bafaloukos, D; Skarlos, D. Weekly paclitaxel as first-line chemotherapy and trastuzumab in patients with advanced breast cancer. A Hellenic

Cooperative Oncology Group phase II study. *Ann Oncol.*, 2001, 12(11), 1545-51.

Freebairn, AJ; Last, AJ; Illidg, TM. Trastuzumab: designer drug or fashionable fad? *Clin Oncol (R Coll Radiol).*, 2001, 13(6), 427-33.

Freebairn, AJ; Last, AJ; Illidg, TM. Trastuzumab: designer drug or fashionable fad? *Clin Oncol (R Coll Radiol).*, 2001, 13(6), 427-33. Review.

Galligioni, E. [Docetaxel (Taxotere) in combination with anthracycline, capecitabin (Xeloda) and new drugs]. *Tumori.*, 2001, 87, (1 Suppl 2), S1-9.

Gerber, B; Krause, A; Markmann, S; Reimer, T; Fietkau, R; Müller, H. Effectiveness of Trastuzumab (Herceptin) in a patient with locally recurrent breast cancer after cardiac failure caused by severe cytotoxic pretreatment. *Oncology.*, 2001, 61(4), 271-4.

Gerber, B; Krause, A; Markmann, S; Reimer, T; Fietkau, R; Müller, H. Effectiveness of Trastuzumab (Herceptin) in a patient with locally recurrent breast cancer after cardiac failure caused by severe cytotoxic pretreatment. *Oncology.*, 2001, 61(4), 271-4.

Gianni, L. Tolerability in patients receiving trastuzumab with or without chemotherapy. *Ann Oncol.*, 2001, 12, Suppl 1, S63-8.

Gillham, CM; Chalmers, AC; Plowman, PN. On the recovery of trastuzumab-related cardiac dysfunction. *Clin Oncol (R Coll Radiol).*, 2001, 13(2), 146.

Goel, S; Mani, S; Perez-Soler, R. Tyrosine kinase inhibitors: a clinical perspective. *Curr Oncol Rep.*, 2002 Jan, 4(1), 9-19.

Goel, S; Mani, S; Perez-Soler, R. Tyrosine kinase inhibitors: a clinical perspective. *Curr Oncol Rep.*, 2002 Jan, 4(1), 9-19.

Guo, S; Wong, S. Cardiovascular toxicities from systemic breast cancer therapy. *Front Oncol.*, 2014, 4, 346.

Guo, S; Wong, S. Cardiovascular toxicities from systemic breast cancer therapy. *Front Oncol.*, 2014, 4, 346.

Hayashi, N; Niikura, N; Masuda, N; Takashima, S; Nakamura, R; Watanabe, K; Kanbayashi, C; Ishida, M; Hozumi, Y; Tsuneizumi, M; Kondo, N; Naito, Y; Honda, Y; Matsui, A; Fujisawa, T; Oshitanai, R;

Yasojima, H; Yamauchi, H; Saji, S; Iwata, H. Prognostic factors of HER2-positive breast cancer patients who develop brain metastasis: a multicenter retrospective analysis. *Breast Cancer Res Treat.*, 2015 149(1), 277-84.

Hayashi, N; Niikura, N; Masuda, N; Takashima, S; Nakamura, R; Watanabe, K; Kanbayashi, C; Ishida, M; Hozumi, Y; Tsuneizumi, M; Kondo, N; Naito, Y; Honda, Y; Matsui, A; Fujisawa, T; Oshitanai, R; Yasojima, H; Yamauchi, H; Saji, S; Iwata, H. Prognostic factors of HER2-positive breast cancer patients who develop brain metastasis: a multicenter retrospective analysis. *Breast Cancer Res Treat.*, 2015, 149(1), 277-84.

Hehl, EM. Opinion on the use of the antitumor drug trastuzumab (Herceptin) in patients with metastatic breast cancer in the county Mecklenburg-Vorpommern. *Int J Clin Pharmacol Ther.*, 2001, 39(11), 503-6.

Hehl, EM. Opinion on the use of the antitumor drug trastuzumab (Herceptin) in patients with metastatic breast cancer in the county Mecklenburg-Vorpommern. *Int J Clin Pharmacol Ther.*, 2001, 39(11), 503-6.

Hortobagyi, GN; Perez, EA. Integration of trastuzumab into adjuvant systemic therapy of breast cancer: ongoing and planned clinical trials. *Semin Oncol.*, 2001, 28, (5 Suppl 16), 41-6.

Hortobagyi, GN. Optimal duration of therapy with trastuzumab. *Semin Oncol.*, 2001, 28, (5 Suppl 16), 33-40.

Hortobagyi, GN. Optimal duration of therapy with trastuzumab. *Semin Oncol.*, 2001, 28, (5 Suppl 16), 33-40.

Hortobagyi, GN. Overview of treatment results with trastuzumab (Herceptin) in metastatic breast cancer. *Semin Oncol.*, 2001, 28, (6 Suppl 18), 43-7.

Huynh, FC; Jones, FE. MicroRNA-7 inhibits multiple oncogenic pathways to suppress HER2Δ16 mediated breast tumorigenesis and reverse trastuzumab resistance. *PLoS One.*, 2014, 9(12), e114419.

Huynh, FC; Jones, FE. MicroRNA-7 inhibits multiple oncogenic pathways to suppress HER2Δ16 mediated breast tumorigenesis and reverse trastuzumab resistance. *PLoS One.*, 2014, 9(12), e114419.

Jakovljevic, M; Gutzwiller, F; Schwenkglenks, M; Milovanovic, O; Rancic, N; Varjacic, M; Stojadinovic, D; Dagovic, A; Matter-Walstra, K. Costs differences among monoclonal antibodies-based first-line oncology cancer protocols for breast cancer, colorectal carcinoma and non-Hodgkin's lymphoma. *J BUON.*, 2014, 19(4), 1111-20.

Jakovljevic, M; Gutzwiller, F; Schwenkglenks, M; Milovanovic, O; Rancic, N; Varjacic, M; Stojadinovic, D; Dagovic, A; Matter-Walstra, K. Costs differences among monoclonal antibodies-based first-line oncology cancer protocols for breast cancer, colorectal carcinoma and non-Hodgkin's lymphoma. *J BUON.*, 2014, 19(4), 1111-20.

Jitawatanarat, P; O'Connor, TL; Kossoff, EB; Levine, EG; Chittawatanarat, K; Ngamphaiboon, N. Safety and tolerability of docetaxel, cyclophosphamide, and trastuzumab compared to standard trastuzumab-based chemotherapy regimens for early-stage human epidermal growth factor receptor 2-positive breast cancer. *J Breast Cancer.*, 2014, 17(4), 356-62.

Jitawatanarat, P; O'Connor, TL; Kossoff, EB; Levine, EG; Chittawatanarat, K; Ngamphaiboon, N. Safety and tolerability of docetaxel, cyclophosphamide, and trastuzumab compared to standard trastuzumab-based chemotherapy regimens for early-stage human epidermal growth factor receptor 2-positive breast cancer. *J Breast Cancer.*, 2014, 17(4), 356-62.

Johnson, PW. The therapeutic use of antibodies for malignancy. *Transfus Clin Biol.*, 2001, 8(3), 255-9.

Jordan, RE; Zhang, N; An, Z. A novel therapeutic strategy to rescue the immune effector function of proteolytically inactivated cancer therapeutic antibodies. *Mol Cancer Ther.*, 2015, 14(3), 681-91.

Jordan, RE; Zhang, N; An, Z. A novel therapeutic strategy to rescue the immune effector function of proteolytically inactivated cancer therapeutic antibodies. *Mol Cancer Ther.*, 2015, 14(3), 681-91.

Kaptain, S; Tan, LK; Chen, B. Her-2/neu and breast cancer. *Diagn Mol Pathol.*, 2001, 10(3), 139-52.

Karagöz, B; Özgün, A; Emirzeoğlu, L; Tunçel, T; Çelik, S; Bilgi, O; Kara, K. Long-term Survival after Lapatinib Rechallenge in Isolated Brain Metastasis of HER2-positive Breast Cancer. *J Breast Health.*, 2015, 11(1), 48-51.

Karagöz, B; Özgün, A; Emirzeoğlu, L; Tunçel, T; Çelik, S; Bilgi, O; Kara, K. Long-term Survival after Lapatinib Rechallenge in Isolated Brain Metastasis of HER2-positive Breast Cancer. *J Breast Health.*, 2015, 11(1), 48-51.

Kim, R; Tanabe, K; Uchida, Y; Osaki, A; Toge, T. The role of HER-2 oncoprotein in drug-sensitivity in breast cancer (review). *Oncol Rep.*, 2002, 9(1), 3-9. Review.

Kim, R; Tanabe, K; Uchida, Y; Osaki, A; Toge, T. The role of HER-2 oncoprotein in drug-sensitivity in breast cancer (review). *Oncol Rep.*, 2002, 9(1), 3-9. Review.

Kobayashi, H; Shirakawa, K; Kawamoto, S; Saga, T; Sato, N; Hiraga, A; Watanabe, I; Heike, Y; Togashi, K; Konishi, J; Brechbiel, MW; Wakasugi, H. Rapid accumulation and internalization of radiolabeled herceptin in an inflammatory breast cancer xenograft with vasculogenic mimicry predicted by the contrast-enhanced dynamic MRI with the macromolecular contrast agent G6-(1B4M-Gd)(256). *Cancer Res.*, 2002, 62(3), 860-6.

Kobayashi, H; Shirakawa, K; Kawamoto, S; Saga, T; Sato, N; Hiraga, A; Watanabe, I; Heike, Y; Togashi, K; Konishi, J; Brechbiel, MW; Wakasugi, H. Rapid accumulation and internalization of radiolabeled herceptin in an inflammatory breast cancer xenograft with vasculogenic mimicry predicted by the contrast-enhanced dynamic MRI with the macromolecular contrast agent G6-(1B4M-Gd)(256). *Cancer Res.*, 2002, 62(3), 860-6.

Kocar, M; Bozkurtlar, E; Telli, F; Serdar Turhal, N; Kaya, H; Kocar, H; Yumuk, F. PTEN loss is not associated with trastuzumab resistance in metastatic breast cancer. *J BUON.*, 2014, 19(4), 900-5.

Kocar, M; Bozkurtlar, E; Telli, F; Serdar Turhal, N; Kaya, H; Kocar, H; Yumuk, F. PTEN loss is not associated with trastuzumab resistance in metastatic breast cancer. *J BUON.*, 2014, 19(4), 900-5.

Konecny, G; Untch, M; Arboleda, J; Wilson, C; Kahlert, S; Boettcher, B; Felber, M; Beryt, M; Lude, S; Hepp, H; Slamon, D; Pegram, M. Her-2/neu and urokinase-type plasminogen activator and its inhibitor in breast cancer. *Clin Cancer Res.*, 2001, 7(8), 2448-57.

Kumamoto, H; Sasano, H; Taniguchi, T; Suzuki, T; Moriya, T; Ichinohasama, R. Chromogenic *in situ* hybridization analysis of HER-2/neu status in breast carcinoma: application in screening of patients for trastuzumab (Herceptin) therapy. *Pathol Int.*, 2001, 51(8), 579-84.

Kumar, R; Yarmand-Bagheri, R. The role of HER2 in angiogenesis. *Semin Oncol.*, 2001, 28(5 Suppl 16), 27-32.

Kumar, R; Yarmand-Bagheri, R. The role of HER2 in angiogenesis. *Semin Oncol.*, 2001, 28(5 Suppl 16), 27-32.

Lane, HA; Motoyama, AB; Beuvink, I; Hynes, NE. Modulation of p27/Cdk2 complex formation through 4D5-mediated inhibition of HER2 receptor signaling. *Ann Oncol.*, 2001, 12, Suppl 1, S21-2.

Latif, Z; Watters, AD; Bartlett, JM; Underwood, MA; Aitchison, M. Gene amplification and overexpression of HER2 in renal cell carcinoma. *BJU Int.*, 2002, 89(1), 5-9.

Latif, Z; Watters, AD; Bartlett, JM; Underwood, MA; Aitchison, M. Gene amplification and overexpression of HER2 in renal cell carcinoma. *BJU Int.*, 2002, 89(1), 5-9.

Leslie, KK. Chemotherapy and pregnancy. *Clin Obstet Gynecol.*, 2002, 45(1), 153-64.

Leslie, KK. Chemotherapy and pregnancy. *Clin Obstet Gynecol.*, 2002, 45(1), 153-64.

Leyland-Jones, B; Arnold, A; Gelmon, K; Verma, S; Ayoub, JP; Seidman, A; Dias, R; Howell, J; Rakhit, A. Pharmacologic insights into the future of trastuzumab. *Ann Oncol.*, 2001, 12, Suppl 1, S43-7.

Leyland-Jones, B; Smith, I. Role of Herceptin in primary breast cancer: views from North America and Europe. *Oncology.*, 2001, 61, Suppl 2, 83-91. Review.

Leyland-Jones, B; Smith, I. Role of Herceptin in primary breast cancer: views from North America and Europe. *Oncology.*, 2001, 61, Suppl 2, 83-91. Review.

Leyland-Jones, B. Dose scheduling--Herceptin. *Oncology.*, 2001, 61, Suppl 2, 31-6.

Li, JW; Mo, M; Yu, KD; Chen, CM; Hu, Z; Hou, YF; Di, GH; Wu, J; Shen, ZZ; Shao, ZM; Liu, GY. ER-poor and HER2-positive: a potential subtype of breast cancer to avoid axillary dissection in node positive patients after neoadjuvant chemo-trastuzumab therapy. *PLoS One.*, 2014, 9(12), e114646.

Li, JW; Mo, M; Yu, KD; Chen, CM; Hu, Z; Hou, YF; Di, GH; Wu, J; Shen, ZZ; Shao, ZM; Liu, GY. ER-poor and HER2-positive: a potential subtype of breast cancer to avoid axillary dissection in node positive patients after neoadjuvant chemo-trastuzumab therapy. *PLoS One.*, 2014, 9(12), e114646.

Li, XJ; Zha, QB; Xu, XY; Xia, L; Zhang, Z; Ren, ZJ; Tang, JH. Lack of prognostic value of human epidermal growth factor-like receptor 2 status in inflammatory breast cancer (IBC): a meta-analysis. *Asian Pac J Cancer Prev.*, 2014, 15(22), 9615-9.

Li, XJ; Zha, QB; Xu, XY; Xia, L; Zhang, Z; Ren, ZJ; Tang, JH. Lack of prognostic value of human epidermal growth factor-like receptor 2 status in inflammatory breast cancer (IBC): a meta-analysis. *Asian Pac J Cancer Prev.*, 2014, 15(22), 9615-9.

Li, ZY; Shan, F; Zhang, LH; Bu, ZD; Wu, AW; Wu, XJ; Zong, XL; Li, SX; Ji, X; Ji, JF. Preoperative chemotherapy with a trastuzumab-containing regimen for a patient with gastric cancer and hepatic metastases. *Genet Mol Res.*, 2014, 13(4), 10952-7.

Li, ZY; Shan, F; Zhang, LH; Bu, ZD; Wu, AW; Wu, XJ; Zong, XL; Li, SX; Ji, X; Ji, JF. Preoperative chemotherapy with a trastuzumab-containing regimen for a patient with gastric cancer and hepatic metastases. *Genet Mol Res.*, 2014, 13(4), 10952-7.

Liu, HL; Gandour-Edwards, R; Lara, PN; Jr. de Vere White, R; LaSalle, JM. Detection of low level HER-2/neu gene amplification in prostate cancer by fluorescence *in situ* hybridization. *Cancer J.*, 2001, 7(5), 395-403.

Livingston, RB; Esteva, FJ. Chemotherapy and herceptin for HER2(+) metastatic breast cancer: the best drug? *Oncologist.*, 2001, 6(4), 315-6.

Lohrisch, C; Piccart, M. An overview of HER2. *Semin Oncol.*, 2001, 28, (6 Suppl 18), 3-11.

Lohrisch, C; Piccart, M. An overview of HER2. *Semin Oncol.*, 2001, 28, (6 Suppl 18), 3-11.

Lu, Y; Zi, X; Zhao, Y; Mascarenhas, D; Pollak, M. Insulin-like growth factor-I receptor signaling and resistance to trastuzumab (Herceptin). *J Natl Cancer Inst.*, 2001, 93(24), 1852-7.

Lu, Y; Zi, X; Zhao, Y; Mascarenhas, D; Pollak, M. Insulin-like growth factor-I receptor signaling and resistance to trastuzumab (Herceptin). *J Natl Cancer Inst.*, 2001, 93(24), 1852-7.

Mann, M; Sheng, H; Shao, J; Williams, CS; Pisacane, PI; Sliwkowski, MX; DuBois, RN. Targeting cyclooxygenase 2 and HER-2/neu pathways inhibits colorectal carcinoma growth. *Gastroenterology.*, 2001, 120(7), 1713-9.

Marano, L; Roviello, F. The distinctive nature of HER2-positive gastric cancers. *Eur J Surg Oncol.*, 2015, 41(3), 271-3.

Marano, L; Roviello, F. The distinctive nature of HER2-positive gastric cancers. *Eur J Surg Oncol.*, 2015, 41(3), 271-3.

Matsumoto, K; Saijo, N. [Issues in cancer treatments--EBM, individuation, and standardization]. *Gan To Kagaku Ryoho.*, 2001, 28(10), 1323-30. Review.

Mayfield, S; Vaughn, JP; Kute, TE. DNA strand breaks and cell cycle perturbation in herceptin treated breast cancer cell lines. *Breast Cancer Res Treat.*, 2001, 70(2), 123-9.

Mayfield, S; Vaughn, JP; Kute, TE. DNA strand breaks and cell cycle perturbation in herceptin treated breast cancer cell lines. *Breast Cancer Res Treat.*, 2001, 70(2), 123-9.

McKeage, K; Perry, CM. Trastuzumab: a review of its use in the treatment of metastatic breast cancer overexpressing HER2. *Drugs.*, 2002, 62(1), 209-43.

McKeage, K; Perry, CM. Trastuzumab: a review of its use in the treatment of metastatic breast cancer overexpressing HER2. *Drugs.*, 2002, 62(1), 209-43.

Meden, H; Beneke, A; Hesse, T; Novophashenny, I; Wischnewsky, M. Weekly intravenous recombinant humanized anti-P185HER2 monoclonal antibody (herceptin) plus docetaxel in patients with metastatic breast cancer: a pilot study. *Anticancer Res.*, 2001, 21(2B), 1301-5.

Ménard, S; Casalini, P; Campiglio, M; Pupa, S; Agresti, R; Tagliabue, E. HER2 overexpression in various tumor types, focussing on its relationship to the development of invasive breast cancer. *Ann Oncol.*, 2001, 12 Suppl, 1, S15-9.

Mendelsohn, J; Baselga, J. The EGF receptor family as targets for cancer therapy. *Oncogene.*, 2000, 19(56), 6550-65.

Miles, DW. Update on HER-2 as a target for cancer therapy: herceptin in the clinical setting. *Breast Cancer Res.*, 2001, 3(6), 380-4.

Miles, DW. Update on HER-2 as a target for cancer therapy: herceptin in the clinical setting. *Breast Cancer Res.*, 2001, 3(6), 380-4.

Miolo, G; Muraro, E; Martorelli, D; Lombardi, D; Scalone, S; Spazzapan, S; Massarut, S; Perin, T; Viel, E; Comaro, E; Talamini, R; Bidoli, E; Turchet, E; Crivellari, D; Dolcetti, R. Anthracycline-free neoadjuvant therapy induces pathological complete responses by exploiting immune proficiency in HER2+ breast cancer patients. *BMC Cancer.*, 2014, 14, 954.

Miolo, G; Muraro, E; Martorelli, D; Lombardi, D; Scalone, S; Spazzapan, S; Massarut, S; Perin, T; Viel, E; Comaro, E; Talamini, R; Bidoli, E; Turchet, E; Crivellari, D; Dolcetti, R. Anthracycline-free neoadjuvant therapy induces pathological complete responses by exploiting immune proficiency in HER2+ breast cancer patients. *BMC Cancer.*, 2014, 14, 954.

Moasser, MM; Basso, A; Averbuch, SD; Rosen, N. The tyrosine kinase inhibitor ZD1839 ("Iressa") inhibits HER2-driven signaling and suppresses the growth of HER2-overexpressing tumor cells. *Cancer Res.*, 2001, 61(19), 7184-8.

Mokbel, K; Elkak, A. Recent advances in breast cancer (the 37th ASCO meeting, May 2001). *Curr Med Res Opin.*, 2001, 17(2), 116-22.

Mokbel, K; Elkak, A. Recent advances in breast cancer (the 37th ASCO meeting, May 2001). *Curr Med Res Opin.*, 2001, 17(2), 116-22.

Mokbel, K; Hassanally, D. From HER2 to herceptin. *Curr Med Res Opin.*, 2001, 17(1), 51-9.

Molina, MA; Codony-Servat, J; Albanell, J; Rojo, F; Arribas, J; Baselga, J. Trastuzumab (herceptin), a humanized anti-Her2 receptor monoclonal antibody, inhibits basal and activated Her2 ectodomain cleavage in breast cancer cells. *Cancer Res.*, 2001, 61(12), 4744-9.

Moore, S. Drug-induced congestive heart failure in breast cancer survivors. *Clin Excell Nurse Pract.*, 2001, 5(3), 129-33.

Moulder, SL; Yakes, FM; Muthuswamy, SK; Bianco, R; Simpson, JF; Arteaga, CL. Epidermal growth factor receptor (HER1) tyrosine kinase inhibitor ZD1839 (Iressa) inhibits HER2/neu (erbB2)-overexpressing breast cancer cells *in vitro* and *in vivo*. *Cancer Res.*, 2001, 61(24), 8887-95.

Moulder, SL; Yakes, FM; Muthuswamy, SK; Bianco, R; Simpson, JF; Arteaga, CL. Epidermal growth factor receptor (HER1) tyrosine kinase inhibitor ZD1839 (Iressa) inhibits HER2/neu (erbB2)-overexpressing breast cancer cells *in vitro* and *in vivo*. *Cancer Res.*, 2001, 61(24), 8887-95.

Mrsić, M; Grgić, M; Budisić, Z; Podolski, P; Bogdanić, V; Labar, B; Jakić-Razumović, J; Restek-Samarzija, N; Gosev, M. Trastuzumab in the treatment of advanced breast cancer: single-center experience. *Ann Oncol.*, 2001, 12 Suppl, 1, S95-6.

Mueller-Holzner, E; Fink, V; Frede, T; Marth, C. Immunohistochemical determination of HER2 expression in breast cancer from core biopsy specimens: a reliable predictor of HER2 status of the whole tumor. *Breast Cancer Res Treat.*, 2001, 69(1), 13-9.

Mueller-Holzner, E; Fink, V; Frede, T; Marth, C. Immunohistochemical determination of HER2 expression in breast cancer from core biopsy specimens: a reliable predictor of HER2 status of the whole tumor. *Breast Cancer Res Treat.*, 2001, 69(1), 13-9.

Neve, RM; Lane, HA; Hynes, NE. The role of overexpressed HER2 in transformation. *Ann Oncol.*, 2001, 12 Suppl 1, S9-13.

Novotný, J; Petruzelka, L; Vedralová, J; Kleibl, Z; Matous, B; Juda, L. Prognostic significance of c-erbB-2 gene expression in pancreatic cancer patients. *Neoplasma.*, 2001, 48(3), 188-91.

Ogura, M. [Adriamycin (doxorubicin)]. *Gan To Kagaku Ryoho.*, 2001 Oct, 28(10), 1331-8. Review.

Ohta, M; Tokuda, Y; Suzuki, Y; Kubota, M; Watanabe, T; Fujii, H; Sasaki, Y; Niwa, T; Makuuchi, H; Tajima, T. A case with HER2-overexpressing breast cancer completely responded to humanized anti-HER2 monoclonal antibody. *Jpn J Clin Oncol.*, 2001, 31(11), 553-6.

Ohta, M; Tokuda, Y; Suzuki, Y; Kubota, M; Watanabe, T; Fujii, H; Sasaki, Y; Niwa, T; Makuuchi, H; Tajima, T. A case with HER2-overexpressing breast cancer completely responded to humanized anti-HER2 monoclonal antibody. *Jpn J Clin Oncol.*, 2001, 31(11), 553-6.

Palmieri, C; Powles, T; Vigushin, D. Trastuzumab and breast cancer. *N Engl J Med.*, 2001, 27, 345(13), 996-7.

Park, JW; Kirpotin, DB; Hong, K; Shalaby, R; Shao, Y; Nielsen, UB; Marks, JD; Papahadjopoulos, D; Benz, CC. Tumor targeting using anti-her2 immunoliposomes. *J Control Release.*, 2001, 74(1-3), 95-113.

Penichet, ML; Dela Cruz, JS; Shin, SU; Morrison, SL. A recombinant IgG3-(IL-2) fusion protein for the treatment of human HER2/neu expressing tumors. *Hum Antibodies.*, 2001, 10(1), 43-9.

Perez, EA; Roche, PC; Jenkins, RB; Reynolds, CA; Halling, KC; Ingle, JN; Wold, LE. HER2 testing in patients with breast cancer: poor correlation between weak positivity by immunohistochemistry and gene amplification by fluorescence *in situ* hybridization. *Mayo Clin Proc.*, 2002, 77(2), 148-54.

Perez, EA; Roche, PC; Jenkins, RB; Reynolds, CA; Halling, KC; Ingle, JN; Wold, LE. HER2 testing in patients with breast cancer: poor correlation between weak positivity by immunohistochemistry and gene amplification by fluorescence *in situ* hybridization. *Mayo Clin Proc.*, 2002, 77(2), 148-54.

Pestalozzi, BC. Correction: Meningeal carcinomatosis from breast carcinoma responsive to trastuzumab. *J Clin Oncol.*, 2001, 19(20), 4091.

Piccart, M; Lohrisch, C; Di Leo, A; Larsimont, D. The predictive value of HER2 in breast cancer. *Oncology.*, 2001, 61 Suppl 2, 73-82.

Piccart, M; Lohrisch, C; Di Leo, A; Larsimont, D. The predictive value of HER2 in breast cancer. *Oncology.*, 2001, 61 Suppl 2, 73-82.

Piccart, MJ. Proposed treatment guidelines for HER2-positive metastatic breast cancer in Europe. *Ann Oncol.*, 2001, 12 Suppl 1, S89-94.

Piechocki, MP; Pilon, SA; Kelly, C; Wei, WZ. Degradation signals in ErbB-2 dictate proteasomal processing and immunogenicity and resist protection by cis glycine-alanine repeat. *Cell Immunol.*, 2001, 212(2), 138-49.

Piechocki, MP; Pilon, SA; Kelly, C; Wei, WZ. Degradation signals in ErbB-2 dictate proteasomal processing and immunogenicity and resist protection by cis glycine-alanine repeat. *Cell Immunol.*, 2001, 212(2), 138-49.

Pienta, KJ. Preclinical mechanisms of action of docetaxel and docetaxel combinations in prostate cancer. *Semin Oncol.*, 2001, 28, (4 Suppl 15), 3-7.

Pierga, JY; Petit, T; Lévy, C; Ferrero, JM; Campone, M; Gligorov, J; Lerebours, F; Roché, H; Bachelot, T; Charafe-Jauffret, E; Bonneterre, J; Hernandez, J; Bidard, FC; Viens, P. Pathological response and circulating tumor cell count identifies treated HER2+ inflammatory breast cancer patients with excellent prognosis: BEVERLY-2 survival data. *Clin Cancer Res.*, 2015, 21(6), 1298-304.

Pierga, JY; Petit, T; Lévy, C; Ferrero, JM; Campone, M; Gligorov, J; Lerebours, F; Roché, H; Bachelot, T; Charafe-Jauffret, E; Bonneterre, J; Hernandez, J; Bidard, FC; Viens, P. Pathological response and circulating tumor cell count identifies treated HER2+ inflammatory breast cancer patients with excellent prognosis: BEVERLY-2 survival data. *Clin Cancer Res.*, 2015, 21(6), 1298-304.

Pircher, M; Mlineritsch, B; Fridrik, MA; Dittrich, C; Lang, A; Petru, E; Weltermann, A; Thaler, J; Hufnagl, C; Gampenrieder, SP;

Rinnerthaler, G; Ressler, S; Ulmer, H; Greil, R. Lapatinib-plus-pegylated liposomal doxorubicin in advanced HER2-positive breast cancer following trastuzumab: a phase II trial. *Anticancer Res.*, 2015, 35(1), 517-21.

Pircher, M; Mlineritsch, B; Fridrik, MA; Dittrich, C; Lang, A; Petru, E; Weltermann, A; Thaler, J; Hufnagl, C; Gampenrieder, SP; Rinnerthaler, G; Ressler, S; Ulmer, H; Greil, R. Lapatinib-plus-pegylated liposomal doxorubicin in advanced HER2-positive breast cancer following trastuzumab: a phase II trial. *Anticancer Res.*, 2015, 35(1), 517-21.

Pivot, X; Manikhas, A; Żurawski, B; Chmielowska, E; Karaszewska, B; Allerton, R; Chan, S; Fabi, A; Bidoli, P; Gori, S; Ciruelos, E; Dank, M; Hornyak, L; Margolin, S; Nusch, A; Parikh, R; Nagi, F; DeSilvio, M; Santillana, S; Swaby, RF; Semiglazov, V. CEREBEL (EGF111438): A Phase III, Randomized, Open-Label Study of Lapatinib Plus Capecitabine Versus Trastuzumab Plus Capecitabine in Patients With Human Epidermal Growth Factor Receptor 2-Positive Metastatic Breast Cancer. *J Clin Oncol.*, 2015, 33(14), 1564-73.

Pivot, X; Manikhas, A; Żurawski, B; Chmielowska, E; Karaszewska, B; Allerton, R; Chan, S; Fabi, A; Bidoli, P; Gori, S; Ciruelos, E; Dank, M; Hornyak, L; Margolin, S; Nusch, A; Parikh, R; Nagi, F; DeSilvio, M; Santillana, S; Swaby, RF; Semiglazov, V. CEREBEL (EGF111438): A Phase III, Randomized, Open-Label Study of Lapatinib Plus Capecitabine Versus Trastuzumab Plus Capecitabine in Patients With Human Epidermal Growth Factor Receptor 2-Positive Metastatic Breast Cancer. *J Clin Oncol.*, 2015, 33(14), 1564-73.

Rubin, I; Yarden, Y. The basic biology of HER2. *Ann Oncol.*, 2001, 12 Suppl 1, S3-8.

Rudlowski, C; Rath, W; Becker, AJ; Wiestler, OD; Buttner, R. Trastuzumab and breast cancer. *N Engl J Med.*, 2001, Sep 27, 345(13), 997-8.

Runowicz, CD. Herceptin: help for advanced breast cancer. *Health News.*, 2001 May, 7(5), 4.

Runowicz, CD. Herceptin: help for advanced breast cancer. *Health News.*, 2001 May, 7(5), 4.

Safran, H; Steinhoff, M; Mangray, S; Rathore, R; King, TC; Chai, L; Berzein, K; Moore, T; Iannitti, D; Reiss, P; Pasquariello, T; Akerman, P; Quirk; D; Mass, R; Goldstein, L; Tantravahi, U. Overexpression of the HER-2/neu oncogene in pancreatic adenocarcinoma. *Am J Clin Oncol.*, 2001 Oct, 24(5), 496-9. Erratum in: *Am J Clin Oncol*, 2002, 25(2), 181.

Savinainen, KJ; Saramäki, OR; Linja, MJ; Bratt, O; Tammela, TL; Isola, JJ; Visakorpi, T. Expression and gene copy number analysis of ERBB2 oncogene in prostate cancer. *Am J Pathol.*, 2002, 160(1), 339-45.

Savinainen, KJ; Saramäki, OR; Linja, MJ; Bratt, O; Tammela, TL; Isola, JJ; Visakorpi, T. Expression and gene copy number analysis of ERBB2 oncogene in prostate cancer. *Am J Pathol.*, 2002, 160(1), 339-45.

Schaller, G; Evers, K; Papadopoulos, S; Ebert, A; Bühler, H. Current use of HER2 tests. *Ann Oncol.*, 2001, 12, Suppl 1, S97-100.

Schneider, JW; Chang, AY; Rocco, TP. Cardiotoxicity in signal transduction therapeutics: erbB2 antibodies and the heart. *Semin Oncol.*, 2001, 28, (5 Suppl 16), 18-26.

Schneider, JW; Chang, AY; Rocco, TP. Cardiotoxicity in signal transduction therapeutics: erbB2 antibodies and the heart. *Semin Oncol.*, 2001, 28, (5 Suppl 16), 18-26.

Scholl, S; Beuzeboc, P; Pouillart, P. Targeting HER2 in other tumor types. *Ann Oncol.*, 2001, 12, Suppl 1, S81-7.

Selcukbiricik, F; Erdamar, S; Buyukunal, E; Serrdengecti, S; Demirelli, F. Is her-2 status in the primary tumor correlated with matched lymph node metastases in patients with gastric cancer undergoing curative gastrectomy? *Asian Pac J Cancer Prev.*, 2014, 15(24), 10607-11.

Selcukbiricik, F; Erdamar, S; Buyukunal, E; Serrdengecti, S; Demirelli, F. Is her-2 status in the primary tumor correlated with matched lymph node metastases in patients with gastric cancer undergoing curative gastrectomy? *Asian Pac J Cancer Prev.*, 2014, 15(24), 10607-11.

Simon, R; Nocito, A; Hübscher, T; Bucher, C; Torhorst, J; Schraml, P; Bubendorf, L; Mihatsch, MM; Moch, H; Wilber, K; Schötzau, A;

Kononen, J; Sauter, G. Patterns of her-2/neu amplification and overexpression in primary and metastatic breast cancer. *J Natl Cancer Inst.*, 2001, 93(15), 1141-6.

Skálová, A; Stárek, Kucerová V; Szépe, P; Plank, L. Salivary duct carcinoma--a highly aggressive salivary gland tumor with HER-2/neu oncoprotein overexpression. *Pathol Res Pract.*, 2001, 197(9), 621-6.

Skopets, IS; Vezikova, NN; Ivanova, EP; Sergeeva, SS; Ignatenko, OV. [A case of irreversible cardiomyopathy induced by polychemotherapy]. *Ter Arkh.*, 2015, 87(12), 73-76.

Skopets, IS; Vezikova, NN; Ivanova, EP; Sergeeva, SS; Ignatenko, OV. [A case of irreversible cardiomyopathy induced by polychemotherapy]. *Ter Arkh.*, 2015, 87(12), 73-76.

Sledge, GW. Jr. Is HER-2/neu a predictor of anthracycline utility? No. *J Natl Cancer Inst Monogr.*, 2001, (30), 85-7.

Sledge, GW. Jr. Is HER-2/neu a predictor of anthracycline utility? No. *J Natl Cancer Inst Monogr.*, 2001, (30), 85-7.

Slichenmyer, WJ; Fry, DW. Anticancer therapy targeting the erbB family of receptor tyrosine kinases. *Semin Oncol.*, 2001, 28, (5 Suppl 16), 67-79.

Slichenmyer, WJ; Fry, DW. Anticancer therapy targeting the erbB family of receptor tyrosine kinases. *Semin Oncol.*, 2001, 28, (5 Suppl 16), 67-79.

Small, EJ; Bok, R; Reese, DM; Sudilovsky, D; Frohlich, M. Docetaxel, estramustine, plus trastuzumab in patients with metastatic androgen-independent prostate cancer. *Semin Oncol.*, 2001, 28, (4 Suppl 15), 71-6.

Smith, I. Future directions in the adjuvant treatment of breast cancer: the role of trastuzumab. *Ann Oncol.*, 2001, 12 Suppl 1, S75-9.

Sorokin, P. New agents and future directions in biotherapy. *Clin J Oncol Nurs.*, 2002, 6(1), 19-24. Review.

Sorokin, P. New agents and future directions in biotherapy. *Clin J Oncol Nurs.*, 2002, 6(1), 19-24. Review.

Strasser, F; Betticher, DC; Suter, TM. Trastuzumab and breast cancer. *N Engl J Med.*, 2001, 345(13), 996.

Sueta, A; Yamamoto, Y; Yamamoto-Ibusuki, M; Hayashi, M; Takeshita, T; Yamamoto, S; Iwase, H. An integrative analysis of PIK3CA mutation, PTEN, and INPP4B expression in terms of trastuzumab efficacy in HER2-positive breast cancer. *PLoS One.*, 2014, 9(12), e116054.

Sueta, A; Yamamoto, Y; Yamamoto-Ibusuki, M; Hayashi, M; Takeshita, T; Yamamoto, S; Iwase, H. An integrative analysis of PIK3CA mutation, PTEN, and INPP4B expression in terms of trastuzumab efficacy in HER2-positive breast cancer. *PLoS One.*, 2014, 9(12), e116054.

Susnjar, S; Bosnjak, S; Radulovic, S. [Trastuzumab in metastatic breast carcinoma]. *Srp Arh Celok Lek.*, 2001, 129(5-6), 147-52.

Susnjar, S; Bosnjak, S; Radulovic, S. [Trastuzumab in metastatic breast carcinoma]. *Srp Arh Celok Lek.*, 2001, 129(5-6), 147-52.

Tan, AR; Swain, SM. Adjuvant chemotherapy for breast cancer: an update. *Semin Oncol.*, 2001, 28(4), 359-76.

Tansi, F; Kallweit, E; Kaether, C; Kappe, K; Schumann, C; Hilger, I; Reissmann, S. Internalization of Near-Infrared Fluorescently Labeled Activatable Cell-Penetrating Peptide and of Proteins into Human Fibrosarcoma Cell Line HT-1080. *J Cell Biochem.*, 2015, 116(7), 1222-31.

Tansi, F; Kallweit, E; Kaether, C; Kappe, K; Schumann, C; Hilger, I; Reissmann, S. Internalization of Near-Infrared Fluorescently Labeled Activatable Cell-Penetrating Peptide and of Proteins into Human Fibrosarcoma Cell Line HT-1080. *J Cell Biochem.*, 2015, 116(7), 1222-31.

Thill, M. New frontiers in oncology: biosimilar monoclonal antibodies for the treatment of breast cancer. *Expert Rev Anticancer Ther.*, 2015, 15(3), 331-8.

Thill, M. New frontiers in oncology: biosimilar monoclonal antibodies for the treatment of breast cancer. *Expert Rev Anticancer Ther.*, 2015, 15(3), 331-8.

Thomson, TA; Hayes, MM; Spinelli, JJ; Hilland, E; Sawrenko, C; Phillips, D; Dupuis, B; Parker, RL. HER-2/neu in breast cancer: interobserver variability and performance of immunohistochemistry with 4 antibodies compared with fluorescent *in situ* hybridization. *Mod Pathol.*, 2001, 14(11), 1079-86.

Thomson, TA; Hayes, MM; Spinelli, JJ; Hilland, E; Sawrenko, C; Phillips, D; Dupuis, B; Parker, RL. HER-2/neu in breast cancer: interobserver variability and performance of immunohistochemistry with 4 antibodies compared with fluorescent *in situ* hybridization. *Mod Pathol.*, 2001, 14(11), 1079-86.

Thor, A. Are patterns of HER-2/neu amplification and expression among primary tumors and regional metastases indicative of those in distant metastases and predictive of Herceptin response? *J Natl Cancer Inst.*, 2001, 93(15), 1120-1.

Tokuda, Y; Suzuki, Y; Ohta, M; Saito, Y; Kubota, M; Tajima, T; Umemura, S; Osamura, RY. Compassionate use of humanized anti-HER2/neu protein, trastuzumab for metastatic breast cancer in Japan. *Breast Cancer.*, 2001, 8(4), 310-5.

Tokuda, Y; Suzuki, Y; Ohta, M; Saito, Y; Kubota, M; Tajima, T; Umemura, S; Osamura, RY. Compassionate use of humanized anti-HER2/neu protein, trastuzumab for metastatic breast cancer in Japan. *Breast Cancer.*, 2001, 8(4), 310-5.

Tsai, KB; Hou, MF; Lin, HJ; Chai, CY; Liu, CS; Huang, TJ. Expression of HER-2/NEU oncoprotein in familial and non-familial breast cancer. *Kaohsiung J Med Sci.*, 2001, 17(2), 64-76.

Umemura, S; Sakamoto, G; Sasano, H; Tsuda, H; Akiyama, F; Kurosumi, M; Tokuda, Y; Watanabe, T; Toi, M; Hasegawa, T; Osamura, RY. Evaluation of HER2 status: for the treatment of metastatic breast cancers by humanized anti-HER2 Monoclonal antibody (trastuzumab) (Pathological committee for optimal use of trastuzumab). *Breast Cancer.*, 2001, 8(4), 316-20.

Umemura, S; Sakamoto, G; Sasano, H; Tsuda, H; Akiyama, F; Kurosumi, M; Tokuda, Y; Watanabe, T; Toi, M; Hasegawa, T; Osamura, RY. Evaluation of HER2 status: for the treatment of metastatic breast cancers by humanized anti-HER2 Monoclonal antibody (trastuzumab)

(Pathological committee for optimal use of trastuzumab). *Breast Cancer.*, 2001, 8(4), 316-20.

Vogel, CL; Cobleigh, MA; Tripathy, D; Gutheil, JC; Harris, LN; Fehrenbacher, L; Slamon, DJ; Murphy, M; Novotny, WF; Burchmore, M; Shak, S; Stewart, SJ. First-line Herceptin monotherapy in metastatic breast cancer. *Oncology.*, 2001, 61, Suppl 2, 37-42.

Vogel, CL; Cobleigh, MA; Tripathy, D; Gutheil, JC; Harris, LN; Fehrenbacher, L; Slamon, DJ; Murphy, M; Novotny, WF; Burchmore, M; Shak, S; Stewart, SJ; Press, M. Efficacy and safety of trastuzumab as a single agent in first-line treatment of HER2-overexpressing metastatic breast cancer. *J Clin Oncol.*, 2002, 20(3), 719-26.

Vogel, CL; Cobleigh, MA; Tripathy, D; Gutheil, JC; Harris, LN; Fehrenbacher, L; Slamon, DJ; Murphy, M; Novotny, WF; Burchmore, M; Shak, S; Stewart, SJ. First-line Herceptin monotherapy in metastatic breast cancer. *Oncology.*, 2001, 61, Suppl 2, 37-42.

Vogel, CL; Cobleigh, MA; Tripathy, D; Gutheil, JC; Harris, LN; Fehrenbacher, L; Slamon, DJ; Murphy, M; Novotny, WF; Burchmore, M; Shak, S; Stewart, SJ; Press, M. Efficacy and safety of trastuzumab as a single agent in first-line treatment of HER2-overexpressing metastatic breast cancer. *J Clin Oncol.*, 2002, 20(3), 719-26.

Waldmann, TA; Levy, R; Coller, BS. Emerging Therapies: Spectrum of Applications of Monoclonal Antibody Therapy. *Hematology Am Soc Hematol Educ Program.*, 2000, 394-408.

Waldmann, TA; Levy, R; Coller, BS. Emerging Therapies: Spectrum of Applications of Monoclonal Antibody Therapy. *Hematology Am Soc Hematol Educ Program.*, 2000, 394-408.

Wang, SC; Zhang, L; Hortobagyi, GN; Hung, MC. Targeting HER2: recent developments and future directions for breast cancer patients. *Semin Oncol.*, 2001, 28, (6 Suppl 18), 21-9.

Wang, SC; Zhang, L; Hortobagyi, GN; Hung, MC. Targeting HER2: recent developments and future directions for breast cancer patients. *Semin Oncol.*, 2001, 28, (6 Suppl 18), 21-9.

Waterhouse, DN; Tardi, PG; Mayer, LD; Bally, MB. A comparison of liposomal formulations of doxorubicin with drug administered in free form: changing toxicity profiles. *Drug Saf.*, 2001, 24(12), 903-20.

Waterhouse, DN; Tardi, PG; Mayer, LD; Bally, MB. A comparison of liposomal formulations of doxorubicin with drug administered in free form: changing toxicity profiles. *Drug Saf.*, 2001, 24(12), 903-20.

Wenzel, C; Schmidinger, M; Huber, H. [Is there progress in chemotherapy for breast cancer?]. *Wien Klin Wochenschr.*, 2001, 113(9), 306-20.

Winer, EP; Burstein, HJ. New combinations with Herceptin in metastatic breast cancer. *Oncology.*, 2001, 61, Suppl 2, 50-7.

Winer, EP; Burstein, HJ. New combinations with Herceptin in metastatic breast cancer. *Oncology.*, 2001, 61, Suppl 2, 50-7.

Wolff, AC. Systemic therapy. *Curr Opin Oncol.*, 2001 Nov, 13(6), 436-49. Review. Erratum in: *Curr Opin Oncol*, 2002 Mar, 14(2), 257.

Wood, WC. Adjuvant therapy for breast cancer: current controversies and future prospects. *J Natl Cancer Inst Monogr.*, 2001, (30), 16.

Wood, WC. Adjuvant therapy for breast cancer: current controversies and future prospects. *J Natl Cancer Inst Monogr.*, 2001, (30), 16.

Xue, J; Jiang, Z; Qi, F; Lv, S; Zhang, S; Wang, T; Zhang, X. Risk of trastuzumab-related cardiotoxicity in early breast cancer patients: a prospective observational study. *J Breast Cancer.*, 2014, 17(4), 363-9.

Xue, J; Jiang, Z; Qi, F; Lv, S; Zhang, S; Wang, T; Zhang, X. Risk of trastuzumab-related cardiotoxicity in early breast cancer patients: a prospective observational study. *J Breast Cancer.*, 2014, 17(4), 363-9.

Yamauchi, H; Stearns, V; Hayes, DF. The Role of c-erbB-2 as a predictive factor in breast cancer. *Breast Cancer.*, 2001, 8(3), 171-83.

Yarden, Y. Biology of HER2 and its importance in breast cancer. *Oncology.*, 2001, 61, Suppl 2, 1-13..

Yip, YL; Ward, RL. Anti-ErbB-2 monoclonal antibodies and ErbB-2-directed vaccines. *Cancer Immunol Immunother.*, 2002, 50(11), 569-87.

Yip, YL; Ward, RL. Anti-ErbB-2 monoclonal antibodies and ErbB-2-directed vaccines. *Cancer Immunol Immunother.*, 2002, 50(11), 569-87.

Yu, AF; Yadav, NU; Lung, BY; Eaton, AA; Thaler, HT; Hudis, CA; Dang, CT; Steingart, RM. Trastuzumab interruption and treatment-induced cardiotoxicity in early HER2-positive breast cancer. *Breast Cancer Res Treat.*, 2015, 149(2), 489-95.

Yu, AF; Yadav, NU; Lung, BY; Eaton, AA; Thaler, HT; Hudis, CA; Dang, CT; Steingart, RM. Trastuzumab interruption and treatment-induced cardiotoxicity in early HER2-positive breast cancer. *Breast Cancer Res Treat.*, 2015, 149(2), 489-95.

Yu, D. Mechanisms of ErbB2-mediated paclitaxel resistance and trastuzumab-mediated paclitaxel sensitization in ErbB2-overexpressing breast cancers. *Semin Oncol.*, 2001, 28, (5 Suppl 16), 12-7.

Yu, D. Mechanisms of ErbB2-mediated paclitaxel resistance and trastuzumab-mediated paclitaxel sensitization in ErbB2-overexpressing breast cancers. *Semin Oncol.*, 2001, 28, (5 Suppl 16), 12-7.

Zulkowski, K; Kath, R; Semrau, R; Merkle, K; Höffken, K. Regression of brain metastases from breast carcinoma after chemotherapy with bendamustine. *J Cancer Res Clin Oncol.*, 2002, 128(2), 111-3.

Zulkowski, K; Kath, R; Semrau, R; Merkle, K; Höffken, K. Regression of brain metastases from breast carcinoma after chemotherapy with bendamustine. *J Cancer Res Clin Oncol.*, 2002, 128(2), 111-3.

Chapter 5

TRASTUZUMAB: INTERACTION WITH OTHER MEDICINAL PRODUCTS

ABSTRACT

Clinically significant interactions between trastuzumab and concomitant medicinal products used in clinical trials will be discussed. The effects of trastuzumab on the pharmacokinetics of other antineoplastic agents will be reviewed.

Keywords: trastuzumab, interactions, drugs, antineoplastic agents

At the end of the 1980s, despite an increase in breast cancer morbidity, a decrease in mortality was recorded. Determination of HER2 gene copy number by FISH may be a more accurate and reliable method for selecting patients eligible for trastuzumab therapy (Tubbs et al., 2001). The main risk factor for breast cancer is gender- breast cancer is one hundred times more common in women than in men. The second important factor increasing the risk of developing breast cancer is age. Breast cancer is rare in women before 30 years of age, about 50% of cases are found in the age group between 50 and 64 years of age, i.e., in the group covered by screening mammography. The basis for the diagnosis of cancer is the result of histopathological examination. Differences in response rates between patients with HER2-overexpressing tumors and those with normal HER2 expression are often (Seidman et al., 2001; Sridhar et al., 2001). The basis of breast cancer treatment is local surgical treatment, mastectomy or conservative therapy with excision of the tumor within the limits of healthy tissues with radiation therapy. Indications for conservative treatment are: cancer stage I or II, the possibility of obtaining a good aesthetic effect and the lack of others medical contraindications. The combination of trastuzumab with adjuvant therapy containing docetaxel and a platinum may provide a helpful alternative to the potentially cardiotoxic trastuzaumab/anthracycline-containing regimens currently under investigation (Pegram et al., 2001; Merimsky et al., 2000; Tokuda et al., 2001). Tumor HER2 status should no longer be ignored because of its direct implications for the optimal management of breast cancer patients (Piccart et al., 2001; Vogel et al., 2001). A fine needle biopsy is performed in patients who are suspected of having metastases in the armpit lymph nodes in physical examination and/or imaging. After confirmation of the metastasis, lymphadenectomy of the axillary lymph nodes is performed. However, if imaging tests reveal no metastases in the armpit lymph nodes, a sentinel node biopsy is performed. In particular, the combination significantly prolonged the median time to disease progression, increased the overall response rate, increased the duration of response, and improved median survival time by approximately 25% compared with chemotherapy alone. The safety profile of trastuzumab either given alone or in combination was favorable (Baselga et al., 2001). To review the standard treatment options for metastatic breast cancer, present recently approved chemotherapeutic and hormonal approaches, and describe novel biologic therapies, particularly the use of monoclonal antibodies. Standard treatment options available to women with metastatic breast cancer include surgery, radiation therapy, hormonal therapy, chemotherapy, and palliative approaches. Trastuzumab, a monoclonal antibody, is a new and promising approach available to a subpopulation of women with metastatic breast cancer (McGinn et al., 2001). The goal of complementary chemotherapy is to reduce the risk of local recurrence and extend the life of patients. The decision on postoperative systemic treatment is taken if the benefits of the therapy outweigh the possible side effects. Individual risk of relapse is determined based on known prognostic factors (tumor size, lymph node involvement, ER expression, PgR, HER2, degree of proliferation, degree of histological malignancy). The patient's general condition, comorbidities, age, menopausal status and the will of the patient are always taken into account. The HER2 oncogene is overexpressed in human pancreatic cancer, but the clinical significance of that overexpression is uncertain. In the present study we investigated the antitumor efficacy of Trastuzumab a new recombinant humanized anti-HER2 antibody, which exhibits cytostatic activity on breast and prostate cancer cells that overexpress the HER2 oncogene. Anthracyclines are antibiotics with high anti-cancer efficacy. The first anthracyclines (doxorubicin and daunorubicin) were synthesized from mushrooms producing the red dye Streptomyces pneucetius. Anthracyclines modify the structure of DNA, among others by the formation of free oxygen radicals in redox reactions. Growth inhibition by trastuzumab was observed in vitro in cell lines with high levels of HER2 expression. Cell lines with low levels of this protein did not respond significantly to the antibody. Two different pancreatic cancer cell lines in an orthotopic mouse model of the disease were studied in vivo (Büchler et al., 2001; Horten et al., 2001; Esteva et al., 2001). Chemotherapy plays an important role in the management of metastatic breast cancer. The anthracyclines (doxorubicin, epirubicin) and the taxanes (paclitaxel, docetaxel) are considered the most active agents for patients with advanced breast cancer. The introduction of taxanes (paclitaxel and docetaxel) for adjuvant treatment of breast cancer with metastases in the armpit lymph nodes prolonged disease-free time and overall survival. Traditionally, the anthracyclines have been used in combination with cyclophosphamide and 5-fluorouracil (FAC, FEC). The taxanes have single-agent activity similar to older combination chemotherapy treatments. There is great interest in developing anthracycline/taxane combinations. Capecitabine is indicated for patients who progress after anthracycline and taxane therapy. Vinorelbine and gemcitabine have activity in patients with metastatic breast cancer and are commonly used as third- and fourth-line palliative therapy. A better understanding of the biology of breast cancer is providing novel treatment approaches. Oncogenes and tumor-supressor genes are emerging as important targets for therapy (Esteva et al., 2001). To determine the true predictive role and strength of the marker for response to each therapy, prospective randomized clinical trials or formal meta-analyses are required (Yamauchi et al., 2001; Burris et al., 2001). In vitro studies have shown that both paclitaxel and docetaxel are responsible for the formation of the toxic metabolite of doxorubicin - doxorubicinol. In the presence of docetaxel, cytosol enzymes are able to metabolize doxorubicinol, while doxorubicin dose reduction is required when combined with paclitaxel and doxorubicin to avoid cardiological complications. Docetaxel is a cytotoxic drug with a similar mechanism of action to paclitaxel, however, a stronger anti-tumor effect associated with, among others with greater affinity for tubulin. Metastatic breast cancer is a partially chemotherapy-sensitive neoplasm. Most chemotherapy groups have activity in this disease, and the most active single drugs are the taxanes, especially docetaxel, and the anthracyclines. The alkylating agents, antimetabolites, and vinca alkaloids are also widely used. Cisplatin appears to be somewhat more active than carboplatin, but direct comparative studies are lacking (Crown et al., 2001). Trastuzumab is a humanized version of the murine monoclonal antibody 4D5. Cardiac toxicity was an unexpected side effect of trastuzumab treatment in the pivotal trials that led to its approval (Sparano et al., 2001). The discovery of the HER2 proto-oncogene and its role in the pathogenesis of breast cancer tumors, and the development of the anti-HER2 monoclonal antibody, trastuzumab, directed against the HER2 receptor represent major milestones in the research developments in breast cancer. Exclusion criteria for the cardiovascular system were: heart failure, ischemic heart disease, poorly controlled hypertension (> 180/100 mmHg), high-risk arrhythmias, and severe valvular disease. In the trastuzumab group, there was a 46% reduction in recurrence risk and fewer deaths. The rationale for the selection of this three-drug regimen is based on the biology of the system and preclinical and clinical findings that demonstrate a high potential for clinical synergy (Slamon et al., 2001). Improvements in breast cancer treatment will arrive with better understanding of its biology and through biologically oriented therapeutic interventions as well as better identification of patient populations susceptible to benefit from classical therapies. Two generations of adjuvant pivotal trials with taxanes have been developed. The first generation compared taxane/anthracycline regimens to nontaxane combinations or sequence regimens. The second generation of trials is presently being performed and contains taxanes in both arms, comparing their use in combination or in sequence. Trastuzumab is the first biologic modifier with significant activity in advanced breast cancer patients amplifying the HER2 gene. As a consequence of these results, including improved survival in the metastatic setting, this agent has been very quickly considered for adjuvant development. However, the significant cardiac toxicity observed with trastuzumab/anthracycline combinations has led to two main strategies for integrating Trastuzumab in the adjuvant setting: (1) addition of Trastuzumab to mostly anthracycline-based programs (sequential approach); and (2) biology-oriented strategy based on synergism between trastuzumab and chemotherapy agents. Large-scale clinical research programs are presently being developed and will create a challenge for clinical researchers. The adequate scientific hypothesis, related to the pivotal studies of trastuzumab in the adjuvant setting, require large sample sizes (several thousand patients) and a very strict selection of the patient population (tumors amplifying the HER2 gene). Success in a timely fashion requires global collaboration, dedication to high-standard clinical research, and awareness of all available protocols by oncologists and patients with breast cancer (Nabholtz et al., 2001; O'Malley et al., 2001, Colomer et al., 2001, (Hellström et al., 2001; Gleiter et al., 2001). The preferred analyses are immunohistochemistry with fluorescent in situ hybridization (FISH) as a follow up test for ambiguous results. Guidelines have been developed for standardized, well controlled procedures for the provision of reliable results. A group of three reference laboratories has been established to provide advice, quality (Ellis et al., 2000). The network is often dysregulated in cancer and lends credence to the mantra that molecular understanding yields clinical benefit (Yarden et al., 2001; Miller et al., 2001). In recent years, the clinical application of paclitaxel (Taxol), docetaxel (Taxotere), vinorelbine (Navelbine), and trastuzumab has improved the management of advanced breast cancer. With the introduction of gemcitabine, a new drug with significant activity in breast cancer has become available. The combination of cisplatin plus gemcitabine is active in relapsed breast cancer patients. The activity observed in drug-resistant patients suggests relative non-cross resistance with other drug combinations (Nagourney et al., 2001; Stern et al., 2000). In clinical practice, the taxanes are now standard therapy in metastatic breast cancer after prior chemotherapy, in particular anthracyclines, has failed (Nabholtz et al., 2000; Eisenhauer et al., 2001; Slamon et al., 2001). Although cardiotoxicity was potentially severe, and in some cases life-threatening, the symptoms generally improved with standard medical management (Chien et al., 2000). HER-2 receptor that is overexpressed, amplified, or both in a number of human malignancies including breast, ovarian, colon, lung, prostate, and cervical cancers. Therefore, a large number of scientists are attempting to control the growth of cancer cells using agents that inhibit one or more of the above steps of growth factor action (Kumar et al., 2000). The epidermal growth factor (also known as HER or ErbB) families of receptor tyrosine kinases are important mediators of cell growth, differentiation, and survival. At present there are 10 ligands that bind directly to epidermal growth factor, HER-3, or HER-4 (Agus et al., 2000). Part of the success of chimeric and humanized antibodies in treating solid tumors relates to the lack of human anti-mouse antibody formation along with enhanced immunogenic effector mechanisms (Murray et al., 2000). Lung cancer, prostate cancer, and ovarian cancer are common epithelial tumors in which clinical trials are currently in progress to explore the potential therapeutic role for monoclonal antibodies to HER2. In preclinical studies with tumor cell lines, trastuzumab was found to have additive and synergistic effects with some chemotherapeutic agents. Clinical trials investigating combination chemotherapy with trastuzumab and a variety of chemotherapeutic agents are already in progress in lung cancer (Agus et al., 2000). HER2 expression may have predictive value regarding response to therapeutic interventions in breast cancer. A number of reports describe the interaction of HER2 overexpression and tamoxifen, but data are inconclusive (Mass, 2000). Metastatic breast carcinoma still remains an incurable condition. The observation of increased antitumor activity between trastuzumab and some chemotherapeutic agents in preclinical models has prompted its use in combination with several drugs (Fornier et al., 2000). Studies with human breast cancer cell lines have shown a causal association between overexpression of the HER-2 proto-oncogene receptor and the acquisition of resistance to tamoxifen. Some clinical studies also indicate that patients with tumors showing high HER-2 levels or high levels of the circulating ectodomain of HER2 may have a lower response to tamoxifen compared with tumors with low HER2 levels or low circulating ectodomain (Nicholson et al., 2000; Perez et al., 2000). In vivo drug/trastuzumab studies were conducted with HER2 transfected MCF7 human breast cancer xenografts in athymic mice. Combinations of trastuzumab plus cisplatin, docetaxel, cyclophosphamide, doxorubicin, paclitaxel, methotrexate, etoposide, and vinblastine in vivo resulted in a significant reduction in xenograft volume compared to chemotherapy-alone controls (Pegram et al., 2000; Schwartz et al., 2000). Amplification of the HER2 gene and overexpression of the HER2 protein induces cell transformation. HER2 overexpression has been suggested to associate with tumor aggressiveness, prognosis and responsiveness to hormonal and cytotoxic agents in breast cancer patients (Kurebayashi et al., 2001). Amplification of the HER2 proto-oncogene has been shown to be accompanied by the overexpression of its protein in the cancer cell membrane (Tsuda et al., 2001; Carter et al., 2001). HER2 is a tyrosine kinase membrane receptor, which when activated, induces a phosphorylation cascade in cytoplasmic kinases leading to increased protein transcription and cellular growth. A high priority for future research is to refine and standardize HER2 testing in order to minimize false-negative results. Furthermore, this procedure would overcome current issues relating to test reproducibility between pathology laboratories and definitions of HER2 positivity (Piccart et al., 2000; Piccart et al., 2001; Vogel et al., 2001). In particular, the combination significantly prolonged the median time to disease progression, increased the overall response rate, increased the duration of response, and improved median survival time by approximately 25% compared with chemotherapy alone. Furthermore, trastuzumab is active as a single agent in women with HER2-positive metastatic breast cancer, inducing durable objective tumor responses. It is of critical importance to standardize the methods used for staining and to apply common interpretation criteria to enable direct comparison of results between laboratories (van de Vijver, 2001; Neve et al., 2001). Similarly, trastuzumab monoclonal antibody combined with chemotherapy prolonged the median time to the progression of breast cancer compared to chemotherapy alone (White et al., 2001; Frankel et al., 2000; Knoop, 2000). Trastuzumab is indicated as a single agent or in combination with chemotherapy for patients with metastatic breast cancer who overexpress the HER2 protein. The toxicity profile of trastuzumab is favorable; cardiac dysfunction has been the primary dose-limiting toxicity, especially when combined with anthracyclines. (Frankel, 2000; Hatanaka et al., 2001). Potential new anticancer agents that target the extracellular ligand-binding region of the receptor include a number of monoclonal antibodies, immunotoxins and ligand-binding cytotoxic agents (Raymond et al., 2000). HER2 is a member of tyrosine kinase growth factor receptor family. On the other hand, a monoclonal antibody, targeting specifically HER2, trastuzumab has been developed and has shown a survival benefit in metastatic breast cancer strongly overexpressing HER2 (Cornez et al., 2000). However, as biologic therapies improve, chemotherapeutic agents are likely to be replaced with biologic agents that are more effective, less toxic, and more patient- and tumor-specific. (Gutheil et al., 2000, Sakamoto et al., 2000; Pittsley et al., 2000; Miller et al., 2000, Scher, 2000; Talukder et al., 2001). Other novel anticancer agents such as paclitaxel, a microtubule binding molecule, and flavopiridol, a cyclin dependent kinase inhibitor, exert their anticancer effects by inhibiting cell cycle progression (Zafonte et al., 2000; Treish et al., 2000). Pharmacogenomic analysis aspires to identify individuals with specific genetic characteristics in order to predict a positive response or reduce a negative response to a therapeutic modality. While the search continues for the many single nucleotide polymorphisms which will be used in such genetic analyses, other genetic alterations in specific cell types have proven useful in determining the potential for response to therapy. One such genetic alteration is amplification of entire gene sequences which results in overexpression of a gene product or protein (Tsongalis et al., 2000). The systemic treatment of breast cancer is a moving target, reflected by the continuous update of treatment guidelines. Chemotherapy regimens, including the adjuvant role of taxanes and preoperative systemic therapy, continue to be optimized. A major challenge facing researchers and clinicians is how to improve the therapeutic index of present and future therapies, identify patients most likely to benefit from the proposed intervention, and avoid treating those who would be exposed to potential toxicities with minimal gain. Anti-estrogens are a prime example of a targeted therapy with a high therapeutic index. Data are now available on aromatase inhibitors in the adjuvant setting and pure antiestrogens in metastatic disease. The role of targeted antihuman epidermal growth factor receptor 2 therapies in the adjuvant setting is being actively investigated, but this is complicated by the inadequate standardization of human epidermal growth factor receptor 2 expression assays used in clinical practice (Wolff et al., 2000). Determination of HER oncogene amplification has become necessary for selection of breast cancer patients for trastuzumab therapy. Fluorescence in situ hybridization (FISH) is currently regarded as a gold standard method for detecting HER2 amplification, but it is not very practical for routine histopathological laboratories. We evaluated a new modification of in situ hybridization, the chromogenic in situ hybridization, which enables detection of HER2 gene copies with conventional peroxidase reaction. Archival formalin-fixed paraffin-embedded tumor tissue sections were pretreated (by heating in a microwave oven and using enzyme digestion) and hybridized with a digoxigenin-labeled DNA probe. The probe was detected with anti-digoxigenin fluorescein, anti-fluorescein peroxidase, and diaminobenzidine (Tanner et al., 2000). Recently there has been resurgence in interest in the use of HER2 protein overexpression or gene amplification to refine prognostic estimates of breast cancer patient outcomes and to predict which therapies might be most appropriate for individual breast cancer patients (Ravdin et al., 2000). Combination studies are not limited to cytotoxic agents, as laboratory and clinical data have demonstrated that HER2 overexpression results in resistance to hormonal therapy. Therefore, a series of studies combining hormonal treatments with trastuzumab is being considered (Baselga et al., 2000). Trastuzumab is not associated with the other commonly observed side effects of chemotherapy, such as alopecia, mucositis, and neutropenia. The results from these studies demonstrate that trastuzumab is active and safe in patients with metastatic HER2-overexpressing breast cancer (Baselga et al., 2000; Pegram et al., 2000; Piccart et al., 2000, Hortobagyi et al., 2000, (Porterfield et al., 2000, McCarthy et al., 2000). A shift toward targeted therapies has also begun, with the incorporation of trastuzumab into the adjuvant setting. Minimizing the long-term toxicity of adjuvant therapy for the large number of women who survive their disease is paramount (McCarthy et al., 2000; McCarthy et al., 2000; Ito, 2000, Mendelsohn, 2000). The use of the monoclonal antibody, trastuzumab, has made specific immunotherapy possible for the first time. The role of high-dose chemotherapy remains uncertain, and further randomized studies are urgently needed (Schmid et al., 2000, Bradbury, 2000; Saijo et al., 2000). The monoclonal antibody trastuzumab, directed against the HER2 protein, has resulted in inhibition of tumor growth in both preclinical and clinical studies. This effect can be increased when used in combination with several chemotherapeutic agents (Gilewski et al., 2000, (Pegram et al., 2000, Brown et al., 2000). These observations provide an immunologic perspective for the use of monoclonal antibody therapy in HER2 protein-receptor-positive breast carcinoma and suggest a role for the clinical laboratory in identifying potential avenues for additional manipulations of the immune system in individual cases in order to enhance the therapeutic response (Brown et al., 2000). The selection of therapies for breast cancer is today based on prognostic features hormone receptor status and HER2 status (trastuzumab therapy) (Hamilton et al., 2000; Scheurle et al., 2000; Marshall et al., 2000, Gottlieb, 2000; Stebbing et al., 2000; Green et al., 2000; Feldman et al., 2000; Hortobagyi et al., 2000). HER2 overexpressing breast cancers may lead to the development of effective biology-based treatment strategies (Yu et al., 2000; Albanell et al., 2000; Keefe, 2000). The pathophysiology of these reactions appears to be secondary to the release of cytokines as the antibodies bind do circulating antigen-expressing cells that are then removed in the reticuloendothelial system of the lungs, spleen and liver (Dillman, 1999, (DeNardo, 1998). Pivotal trials in breast cancer showed that it has activity as a single agent in a subset of patients whose tumors greatly over-express HER2, but results were even more impressive when it was used in combination with chemotherapy. It should also prove to be useful in the treatment of subsets of patients with other adenocarcinomas whose tumors over-express HER2 (Dillman, 1999; Cohen, 1999; Mandler et al., 2000; Pestalozzi et al., 2000; Burris et al., 2000; Noonberg et al., 2000, McNeil, 2000, Perez, 1999; Perez, 1999). Mouse monoclonal antibodies, as well as the humanized, clinically effective therapeutic agents trastuzumab and rituximab, engaged both activation and inhibitory antibody receptors on myeloid cells, thus modulating their cytotoxic potential (Clynes et al., 2000, (Houghton et al., 2000, (Titus, 1999, (Persons et al., 2000; Persons et al., 2000). Clinical activity with one of these antibodies, trastuzumab, a humanized anti-ErbB2 MAb, has been documented in patients with breast cancer in a series of clinical trials and has recently been approved for the therapy of patients with metastatic ErbB2 overexpressing breast cancer. In addition to antibodies, compounds that inhibit receptor tyrosine kinases have shown significant preclinical activity and are currently being evaluated in the clini c (Albanell et al., 1999, (Nelson, 2000). As new anthracycline/taxane combinations establish themselves in earlier stages of the disease, the need for effective, non-cross resistant salvage regimens will emerge (Lebwohl et al., 1999, (Nelson, 2000, Lebwohl et al., 2000). HER2 was precise and resistant to interferences, characteristics that are essential for longitudinal monitoring of cancer patients (Payne et al., 2000; Park et al., 2000). Evaluation of the efficacy of trastuzumab in Her2 overexpressors with carcinoma of unknown primary site is indicated (Hainsworth et al., 2000, Stephenson, 2000; Holm-Hansen et al., 2000). These findings indicate that combined treatment with anti-HER2 antibody and anti-oestrogen may be useful for the treatment of patients with breast cancer expressing both ER and HER2 (Kunisue et al., 2000;

Kollmannsberger et al., 1999). Herceptin results in significant antitumor activity with the potential for reducing toxicity in metastatic breast cancer patients (Colbern et al., 1999, (Nissenblatt et al., 1999). Such a therapeutic approach has already been found effective in experimental tumor models and in clinical trials as well. Further understanding of the importance of erbB2 and growth factor receptors in the transformation of normal cells to malignant ones may once give us a chance to cure erbB2 over-expressing breast cancer (Nagy et al., 1999; Tokuda et al., 1999; Sporn et al., 1999). Shortly after treatment with the cytostatic combination of cisplatin and paclitaxel was generally accepted as the standard therapy for patients with epithelial ovarian carcinoma, many have come to regard the combination of carboplatin and paclitaxel as a better choice (Sibbald et al., 1999; Weiner, 1999). These exciting results provide a basis for further refinement of the existing approaches to develop new antibody-based cancer therapy strategies (Penault-Llorca et al., 1999; Marshall et al., 1999). Recent advances in understanding how response or resistance to cytotoxic drugs develops at the cellular level resulted in the development of novel, non-cytotoxic agents that modulate response the chemotherapy. Clinical experience with the anti-HER2 antibody, trastuzumab, in breast cancer has demonstrated that manipulation of growth factor signalling can enhance sensitivity to cytotoxic drugs in a clinically meaningful way. (Pusztai et al., 1999; Mordenti et al., 1999; Agus et al., 1999). Treatment of advanced breast cancer with autologous stem cell transplantation is limited by a high probability of disease relapse (Cooley et al., 1999; Ravdin, 1999). Approaches for additional study of the extent and severity of trastuzumab cardiotoxicity are briefly addressed (Ewer et al., 1999). Such receptor-enhanced chemosensitivity offers a new approach to target overexpressed growth factor receptors in a variety of cancers, which will lead to new, biologically based therapeutic strategies for clinical intervention (Pegram et al., 1999). These results suggest that trastuzumab may be associated with an amelioration of the deleterious effects of chemotherapy alone. In summary, in the doses and schedules used in these studies, trastuzumab is not associated with worsening of HRQL (Osoba et al., 1999). Minor responses, seen in two patients, and stable disease, which occurred in 14 patients, lasted for a median of 5.1 months (Baselga et al., 1999; Shak, 1999). The HER2 system, enlists immune cells to attack and kill the tumor target, and augmenting chemotherapy-induced cytotoxicity (Sliwkowski et al., 1999). Conjugates composed of anti-CD33 antibodies and the chemotherapy agent, calicheamicin, show promising activity in patients with relapsed or refractory acute myelogenous leukemia. Treatment of patients with advanced breast cancer using the anti-HER2/neu antibody trastuzumab leads to objective responses in some patients whose tumors overexpress the HER2/neu oncoprotein. These exciting results justify recent enthusiasm for continued efforts to refine existing approaches and to develop new antibody-based strategies to treat human malignancy (Weiner, 1999). Although there is no rigid standard for the sequencing of therapy for management of metastatic breast cancer, chemotherapy has a role in the treatment program for nearly all patients with this disease. The goal of treatment remains meaningful palliation of patients with complications of progressive cancer (Perez, 1999). The effectiveness and negligible side-effects of the chimeric antibody against HER2 (Herceptin) render it a valuable tool in the treatment of breast cancer (Schaller et al., 1999; Ye et al., 1999). The HER2 oncogene has been extensively investigated as a prognostic factor and recently as a predictor of response to chemotherapy or endocrine therapy. The development of a humanized anti-HER-2 monoclonal antibody (Herceptin) and the encouraging results obtained in the treatment of patients with HER-2 overexpressing metastatic breast cancer with this antibody have resulted in renewed interest in HER2. This article reviews the current knowledge of HER2 both as a prognostic and a predictive factor. Problems associated with the standardization of the methodology for assessing HER2 status and clinically significant cut-off points are addressed (Hanna et al., 1999, (Roche et al., 1999). The development of additional docetaxel combinations, schedules, and regimens as a result of the newly available therapies in the management of breast cancer holds promise for the future (Hortobagyi et al., 1999; Hussar, 1999; Beuzeboc et al., 1999; Glaser, 1999; Perez, 1998). The use of paclitaxel on a weekly schedule or with new therapeutic modalities, such as monoclonal antibodies, is also receiving much attention. While it is clear that paclitaxel is a very active agent in the treatment of breast cancer, it is hoped that these innovative trials will further maximize the potential of this agent in patients with breast cancer (Perez, 1998). The potential role of new aromatase inhibitors as first-line hormonal agents requires further study. Finally, the possible synergy between trastuzumab, a recombinant humanized monoclonal antibody to the HER-2/neu protein, and paclitaxel (Taxol) is being studied in two clinical trials (Fornier et al., 1999, (Valgus, 1999, Check, 1999; Vogel et al., 1999; Jerian et al., 1999). The synergistic interaction of HER2 with alkylating agents, platinum analogs and topoisomerase II inhibitors, as well as the additive interaction with taxanes, anthracyclines and some antimetabolites in HER-2 overexpressing breast cancer cells demonstrates that these are rational combinations to test in human clinical trials (Pegram et al., 1999; Goldenberg, 1999; Norton, 1999; Workman, 1999; Brenner et al., 1999; Wisecarver, 1999). The difficulty in comparing results from different data sets due to the wide variety of reagents and technologies used to detect HER2 amplification/overexpression in clinical specimens is also discussed. Finally, we report results from experimental models of HER2 overexpression which have been used in an effort to understand the relationship between HER2 and response to chemotherapeutics and antiestrogens in breast cancer (Pegram et al., 1998; McNeil, 1999; Wong, 1999; Haseltine, 1998; Miller, 1998; Butera et al., 1998; Mabro, 1998; Graziano, 1998; Pegram et al., 1998; Eiermann, 1998, Nass et al., 1998; Baselga et al., 1998). Recombinant humanized anti-HER2 antibody inhibits the growth of breast cancer cells overexpressing HER2 and has clinical activity (Garratt et al., 2003; Zhu et al., 2002; Haller, 2002; Montemurro et al., 2003; Colón et al., 2002; Colón et al., 2002; Jalava et al., 2002; Bookman et al., 2003). Through a phosphatidylinositol 3'-kinase-dependent pathway, HER2 stimulates the FAS promoter and ultimately mediates increased fatty acid synthesis (Geffen et al., 2002; Burstein et al., 2003; Camirand et al., 2002; Longo et al., 2002; Clark et al., 2002; Wu et al., 2002; Laban et al., 2003). Cardiac complications during adjuvant treatment with trastuzumab that resulted in discontinuation of treatment in the study group were transient. This may indicate the advisability of continuing adjuvant trastuzumab therapy. In adjuvant treatment, the recommended total dose of anthracyclines should not be exceeded, as this is associated with an increased risk of cardiac complications. An increased risk of cardiotoxicity during adjuvant trastuzumab therapy was found in patients with hypertension, ischemic heart disease, hypothyroidism and heavy smokers - these patients require special cardiological supervision.

ACKNOWLEDGMENTS

Dorota Bartusik-Aebisher acknowledges support from the National Center of Science NCN (New drug delivery systems-MRI study, Grant OPUS-13 number 2017/25/B/ST4/02481).

REFERENCES

Agus DB, Akita RW, Fox WD, Lofgren JA, Higgins B, Maiese K, Scher HI, Sliwkowski MX. A potential role for activated HER-2 in prostate cancer. *Semin Oncol.* 2000;27(6 Suppl 11):76-83; discussion 92-100.

Agus DB, Bunn PA Jr, Franklin W, Garcia M, Ozols RF. HER-2/neu as a therapeutic target in non-small cell lung cancer, prostate cancer, and ovarian cancer. *Semin Oncol.* 2000;27(6 Suppl 11):53-63; discussion 92-100.

Agus DB, Scher HI, Higgins B, Fox WD, Heller G, Fazzari M, Cordon-Cardo C, Golde DW. Response of prostate cancer to anti-Her-2/neu antibody in androgen-dependent and -independent human xenograft models. *Cancer Res.* 1999;59(19):4761-4.

Albanell J, Baselga J. Systemic therapy emergencies. *Semin Oncol.* 2000 Jun;27(3):347-61.

Albanell J, Baselga J. The ErbB receptors as targets for breast cancer therapy. *J Mammary Gland Biol Neoplasia.* 1999;4(4):337-51.

Barnes DM, Miles DW. Response of metastatic breast cancer to trastuzumab? *Lancet.* 2000; 355(9199):160-1.

Baselga J, Norton L, Albanell J, Kim YM, Mendelsohn J. Recombinant humanized anti-HER2 antibody (Herceptin) enhances the antitumor activity of paclitaxel and doxorubicin against HER2/neu overexpressing human breast cancer xenografts. *Cancer Res.* 1998; 58(13): 2825-31.

Baselga J, Tripathy D, Mendelsohn J, Baughman S, Benz CC, Dantis L, Sklarin NT, Seidman AD, Hudis CA, Moore J, Rosen PP, Twaddell T, Henderson IC, Norton L. Phase II study of weekly intravenous trastuzumab (Herceptin) in patients with HER2/neu-overexpressing metastatic breast cancer. *Semin Oncol.* 1999;26(4 Suppl 12):78-83.

Baselga J. Clinical trials of Herceptin(R) (trastuzumab). *Eur J Cancer.* 2001;37 Suppl 1:18-24.

Baselga J. Clinical trials of single-agent trastuzumab (Herceptin). *Semin Oncol.* 2000;27(5 Suppl 9):20-6.

Baselga J. Current and planned clinical trials with trastuzumab (Herceptin). *Semin Oncol.* 2000; 27(5 Suppl 9):27-32.

Beuzeboc P, Scholl S, Garau XS, Vincent-Salomon A, Cremoux PD, Couturier J, Palangié T, Pouillart P. [Herceptin, a monoclonal humanized antibody anti-HER2: a major therapeutic progress in breast cancers overexpressing this oncogene? *Bull Cancer.* 1999;86(6):544-9.

Bookman MA, Darcy KM, Clarke-Pearson D, Boothby RA, Horowitz IR. Evaluation of monoclonal humanized anti-HER2 antibody, trastuzumab, in patients with recurrent or refractory ovarian or primary peritoneal carcinoma with overexpression of HER2: a phase II trial of the Gynecologic Oncology Group. *J Clin Oncol.* 2003;21(2):283-90.

Bradbury J. Vaccine against breast and ovarian cancer still on the horizon. *Mol Med Today.* 2000;6(10):378.

Brenner TL, Adams VR. First MAb approved for treatment of metastatic breast cancer. *J Am Pharm Assoc* (Wash). 1999;39(2):236-8. Review.

Bridges AJ. The rationale and strategy used to develop a series of highly potent, irreversible, inhibitors of the epidermal growth factor receptor family of tyrosine kinases. *Curr Med Chem.* 1999;6(9):825-43.

Brown RE, Bernath AM, Lewis GO. HER-2/neu protein-receptor-positive breast carcinoma: an immunologic perspective. *Ann Clin Lab Sci.* 2000;30(3):249-58.

Büchler P, Reber HA, Büchler MC, Roth MA, Büchler MW, Friess H, Isacoff WH, Hines OJ. Therapy for pancreatic cancer with a recombinant humanized anti-HER2 antibody (herceptin). *J Gastrointest Surg.* 2001;5(2):139-46.

Burris HA 3rd. Docetaxel (Taxotere) in HER-2-positive patients and in combination with trastuzumab (Herceptin). *Semin Oncol.* 2000;27(2 Suppl 3):19-23.

Burris HA 3rd. Docetaxel (Taxotere) plus trastuzumab (Herceptin) in breast cancer. *Semin Oncol.* 2001;28(1 Suppl 3):38-44.

Burstein HJ, Harris LN, Gelman R, Lester SC, Nunes RA, Kaelin CM, Parker LM, Ellisen LW, Kuter I, Gadd MA, Christian RL, Kennedy PR, Borges VF, Bunnell CA, Younger J, Smith BL, Winer EP. Preoperative therapy with trastuzumab and paclitaxel followed by sequential adjuvant doxorubicin/cyclophosphamide for HER2 overexpressing stage II or III breast cancer: a pilot study. *J Clin Oncol.* 2003;21(1):46-53.

Butera J, Malachovsky M, Rathore R, Safran H. Novel approaches in development for the treatment of pancreatic cancer. *Front Biosci.* 1998;3:E226-9.

Camirand A, Lu Y, Pollak M. Co-targeting HER2/ErbB2 and insulin-like growth factor-1 receptors causes synergistic inhibition of growth in HER2-overexpressing breast cancer cells. *Med Sci Monit.* 2002;8(12):BR521-6.

Carter WB, Hoying JB, Boswell C, Williams SK. HER2/neu overexpression induces endothelial cell retraction. *Int J Cancer.* 2001;91(3):295-9.

Chan KC, Knox WF, Gandhi A, Slamon DJ, Potten CS, Bundred NJ. Blockade of growth factor receptors in ductal carcinoma in situ inhibits epithelial proliferation. *Br J Surg.* 2001; 88(3):412-8.

Check W. More than one way to look for HER2. *CAP Today.* 1999;13(3):1, 40-2, 46,

Chien KR. Myocyte survival pathways and cardiomyopathy: implications for trastuzumab cardiotoxicity. *Semin Oncol.* 2000;27(6 Suppl 11):9-14; 92-100. Review.

Clark AS, West K, Streicher S, Dennis PA. Constitutive and inducible Akt activity promotes resistance to chemotherapy, trastuzumab, or tamoxifen in breast cancer cells. Mol Cancer Ther. 2002;1(9):707-17.

Clynes RA, Towers TL, Presta LG, Ravetch JV. Inhibitory Fc receptors modulate in vivo cytotoxicity against tumor targets. Nat Med. 2000;6(4):443-6.

Cohen RL. Herceptin: breaking new ground. *Cancer Biother Radiopharm.* 1999;14(1):1-4. No abstract available.

Colbern GT, Hiller AJ, Musterer RS, Working PK, Henderson IC. Antitumor activity of Herceptin in combination with STEALTH liposomal cisplatin or nonliposomal cisplatin in a HER2 positive human breast cancer model. *J Inorg Biochem.* 1999;77(1-2):117-20.

Colomer R, Shamon LA, Tsai MS, Lupu R. Herceptin: from the bench to the clinic. *Cancer Invest.* 2001;19(1):49-56. Review. No abstract available.

Colón E, Reyes JS, González Keelan C, Climent-Peris C. Prevalence of steroid receptors and HER 2/neu in breast cancer biopsies of women living in Puerto Rico. *P R Health Sci J.* 2002 Dec;21(4):299-303.

Cooley S, Burns LJ, Repka T, Miller JS. Natural killer cell cytotoxicity of breast cancer targets is enhanced by two distinct mechanisms of antibody-dependent cellular cytotoxicity against LFA-3 and HER2/neu. *Exp Hematol.* 1999;27(10):1533-41.

Cornez N, Piccart MJ. [Breast cancer and herceptin]. *Bull Cancer.* 2000;87(11):847-58. Review. French.

Cox G, Vyberg M, Melgaard B, Askaa J, Oster A, O'Byrne KJ. Herceptest: HER2 expression and gene amplification in non-small cell lung cancer. *Int J Cancer.* 2001; 92(4):480-3.

Crown JP. The platinum agents: a role in breast cancer treatment? *Semin Oncol.* 2001;28(1 Suppl 3):28-37. Review.

DeNardo GL. Biotherapy of cancer marches on! *Cancer Biother Radiopharm.* 1998; 13(5):335-6. No abstract available.

Dillman RO. Infusion reactions associated with the therapeutic use of monoclonal antibodies in the treatment of malignancy. *Cancer Metastasis Rev.* 1999;18(4):465-71. Review.

Dillman RO. Perceptions of Herceptin: a monoclonal antibody for the treatment of breast cancer. *Cancer Biother Radiopharm.* 1999;14(1):5-10. Review.

Eiermann W. [New antibody for breast cancer therapy. Interview by Brigitte Schalhorn]. *Fortschr Med.* 1998 Jun 30;116(18-19):18. German. No abstract available.

Eisenhauer EA. From the molecule to the clinic--inhibiting HER2 to treat breast cancer. *N Engl J Med.* 2001;344(11):841-2. No abstract available.

Ellis IO, Dowsett M, Bartlett J, Walker R, Cooke T, Gullick W, Gusterson B, Mallon E, Lee PB. Recommendations for HER2 testing in the UK. *J Clin Pathol. 2000*;53(12):890-2.

Esteva FJ, Valero V, Pusztai L, Boehnke-Michaud L, Buzdar AU, Hortobagyi GN. Chemotherapy of metastatic breast cancer: what to expect in 2001 and beyond. *Oncologist.* 2001;6(2):133-46. Review.

Ewer MS, Gibbs HR, Swafford J, Benjamin RS. Cardiotoxicity in patients receiving transtuzumab (Herceptin): primary toxicity, synergistic or sequential stress, or surveillance artifact? *Semin Oncol.* 1999;26(4 Suppl 12):96-101.

Feldman AM, Lorell BH, Reis SE. Trastuzumab in the treatment of metastatic breast cancer: anticancer therapy versus cardiotoxicity. *Circulation.* 2000;102(3):272-4. Review.

Fischman J. On target. A new generation of drugs offers customized cures. *US News World Rep.* 2003;134(2):50-2, 55-6, 58. No abstract available.

Fleming TR. Issues in the design of clinical trials: insights from the trastuzumab (Herceptin) experience. *Semin Oncol.* 1999;26(4 Suppl 12):102-7.

Fornier M, Esteva FJ, Seidman AD. Trastuzumab in combination with chemotherapy for the treatment of metastatic breast cancer. *Semin Oncol.* 2000;27(6 Suppl 11):38-45; discussion 92-100.

Fornier M, Munster P, Seidman AD. Update on the management of advanced breast cancer. *Oncology* (Williston Park). 1999;13(5):647-58; discussion 660, 663-4.

Frankel C. Development and clinical overview of trastuzumab (herceptin). *Semin Oncol Nurs.* 2000;16(4 Suppl 1):13-7.

Frankel C. Nursing management considerations with trastuzumab (herceptin). *Semin Oncol Nurs.* 2000;16(4 Suppl 1):23-8.

Garratt AN, Ozcelik C, Birchmeier C. ErbB2 pathways in heart and neural diseases. *Trends Cardiovasc Med.* 2003;13(2):80-6.

Geffen DB, Man S. New drugs for the treatment of cancer, 1990-2001. *Isr Med Assoc J.* 2002; 4(12):1124-31.

Gilewski T, Seidman A, Norton L, Hudis C. An immunotherapeutic approach to treatment of breast cancer: focus on trastuzumab plus paclitaxel. Breast Cancer Medicine Service. *Cancer Chemother Pharmacol.* 2000;46 Suppl:S23-6.

Glaser V. Genentech relaunched with independence intact. *Nat Biotechnol.* 1999;17(7):634.

Gleiter S, Lilie H. Coupling of antibodies via protein Z on modified polyoma virus-like particles. *Protein Sci.* 2001;10(2):434-44.

Goldenberg MM. Trastuzumab, a recombinant DNA-derived humanized monoclonal antibody, a novel agent for the treatment of metastatic breast cancer. *Clin Ther.* 1999;21(2):309-18. Review.

Gottlieb S. Cancer drug may cause heart failure. *BMJ.* 2000; 321(7256):259.

Graziano C. HER-2 breast assay, linked to Herceptin, wins FDA's okay. *CAP Today.* 1998; 12(10):1, 14-6. No abstract available.

Green MC, Murray JL, Hortobagyi GN. Monoclonal antibody therapy for solid tumors. *Cancer Treat Rev.* 2000;26(4):269-86.

Gutheil JC. Novel immunologic and biologic therapies for breast cancer. *Curr Oncol Rep.* 2000; 2(6):582-6.

Haller DG. Future directions in the treatment of pancreatic cancer. *Semin Oncol.* 2002;29(6 Suppl 20):31-9.

Hainsworth JD, Lennington WJ, Greco FA. *Overexpression of Her-2 in patients with poorly differentiated carcinoma or poorly differentiated adenocarcinoma of unknown primary site.*

Hamilton A, Piccart M. The contribution of molecular markers to the prediction of response in the treatment of breast cancer: a review of the literature on HER-2, p53 and BCL-2. *Ann Oncol.* 2000;11(6):647-63.

Hanna W, Kahn HJ, Trudeau M. Evaluation of HER-2/neu (erbB-2) status in breast cancer: from bench to bedside. *Mod Pathol.* 1999;12(8):827-34.

Haseltine WA. Not quite pharmacogenomics. *Nat Biotechnol.* 1998;16(13):1295.

Hatanaka Y, Hashizume K, Kamihara Y, Itoh H, Tsuda H, Osamura RY, Tani Y. Quantitative immunohistochemical evaluation of HER2/neu expression with HercepTestTM in breast carcinoma by image analysis. *Pathol Int.* 2001;51(1):33-6.

Heinzl S. [Trastuzumab. Monoclonal antibody for the treatment of breast cancer]. *Med Monatsschr Pharm.* 2000;23(11):350-2.

Hellström I, Goodman G, Pullman J, Yang Y, Hellström KE. Overexpression of HER-2 in ovarian carcinomas. *Cancer Res.* 2001;61(6):2420-3.

Horten B, Da Silva M, Thompson J. HER2 testing. *CAP Today.* 2001;15(1):8-9.

Hortobagyi GN, Khayat D. Targeting progress: the development of growth factor receptor-directed therapy. *Semin Oncol.* 2000;27(5 Suppl 9):1-2.

Hortobagyi GN. Developments in chemotherapy of breast cancer. *Cancer.* 2000;88(12 Suppl):3073-9.

Hortobagyi GN. Recent progress in the clinical development of docetaxel (Taxotere). *Semin Oncol.* 1999;26(3 Suppl 9):32-6.

Horton J. Trastuzumab use in breast cancer: clinical issues. *Cancer Control.* 2002-Dec;9(6):499-507..

Houghton AN, Scheinberg DA. Monoclonal antibody therapies-a 'constant' threat to cancer. *Nat Med.* 2000;6(4):373-4.

Hussar DA. *New drugs 99,* Part III. Nursing. 1999;29(6):43-7.

Ito Y. [Paclitaxel for treatment of advanced breast cancers]. *Nihon Rinsho.* 2000 Apr;58 Suppl:259-64.

Jalava PJ, Kuopio T, Kortelainen S, Kronqvist P, Collan YU. Quantitation of erbB2 positivity for evaluation of high-risk patients. *Ann Med.* 2002;34(7-8):544-53.

Jerian S, Keegan P. Cardiotoxicity associated with paclitaxel/trastuzumab combination therapy. *J Clin Oncol.* 1999;17(5):1647-8.

Keefe DL. Cardiovascular emergencies in the cancer patient. *Semin Oncol.* 2000;27(3):244-55.

Knoop T. Educational and psychosocial issues related to new treatment advances for metastatic breast cancer. *Semin Oncol Nurs.* 2000;16(4 Suppl 1):18-22.

Kollmannsberger C, Pressler H, Mayer F, Kanz L, Bokemeyer C. Cisplatin-refractory, HER2/neu-expressing germ-cell cancer: induction of remission by the monoclonal antibody Trastuzumab. *Ann Oncol.* 1999;10(11):1393-4.

Konecny G, Slamon DJ. HER2 testing and correlation with efficacy of trastuzumab therapy. *Oncology* (Williston Park). 2002;16(11):1576, 1578.

Kumar R, Mandal M, Vadlamudi R. New insights into anti-HER-2 receptor monoclonal antibody research. *Semin Oncol.* 2000;27(6 Suppl 11):84-91;

Kumar-Sinha C, Ignatoski KW, Lippman ME, Ethier SP, Chinnaiyan AM. Transcriptome analysis of HER2 reveals a molecular connection to fatty acid synthesis. *Cancer Res.* 2003;63(1):132-9.

Kunisue H, Kurebayashi J, Otsuki T, Tang CK, Kurosumi M, Yamamoto S, Tanaka K, Doihara H, Shimizu N, Sonoo H. Anti-HER2 antibody enhances the growth inhibitory effect of anti-oestrogen on breast cancer cells expressing both oestrogen receptors and HER2. *Br J Cancer.* 2000;82(1):46-51.

Kurebayashi J. Biological and clinical significance of HER2 overexpression in breast cancer. *Breast Cancer.* 2001;8(1):45-51.

Laban C, Bustin SA, Jenkins PJ. The GH-IGF-I axis and breast cancer. *Trends Endocrinol Metab.* 2003;14(1):28-34.

Lebwohl DE, Canetta R. New developments in chemotherapy of advanced breast cancer. *Ann Oncol.* 1999;10 Suppl 6:139-46.

Longo F, Mansueto G. [Breast Cancer Conference. Trastuzumab and capecitabine in the treatment of advanced breast cancer. Milano, 6-7 June 2002]. *Tumori.* 2002;88(5):A1-10.

Longo F, Mansueto G. [National Conference of Medical Oncology. New trends in cancer therapy. Genova, October 29, 2000]. *Tumori.* 2000;86(6):A5-12.

Lück HJ, Roché H. Weekly paclitaxel: an effective and well-tolerated treatment in patients with advanced breast cancer. *Crit Rev Oncol Hematol.* 2002;44 Suppl:S15-30.

Mabro M. [Cancerology: search for better therapeutic schemes]. *Presse Med.* 1998;27(24):1228-30.

Mandler R, Dadachova E, Brechbiel JK, Waldmann TA, Brechbiel MW. Synthesis and evaluation of antiproliferative activity of a geldanamycin-Herceptin immunoconjugate. *Bioorg Med Chem Lett.* 2000;10(10):1025-8.

Marshall E. Oncologist encouraged by cancer advance. Dr. Blachly steps up the case for breast cancer screening. *J Ark Med Soc.* 1999 Oct;96(5):174-5. No abstract available.

Marshall E. Patent disputes. Biotech giants butt heads over cancer drug. *Science.* 2000;288(5475):2303.

Mass R. The role of HER-2 expression in predicting response to therapy in breast cancer. *Semin Oncol.* 2000;27(6 Suppl 11):46-52;

McCarthy NJ, Swain SM. Update on adjuvant chemotherapy for early breast cancer. Oncology (Williston Park). 2000 Sep;14(9):1267-80; discussion 1280-4, 1287-8. Review. *Erratum in: Oncology* (Huntingt) 2000;14(12):1697.

McGinn K, Moore J. Metastatic breast cancer: understanding current management options. Oncol Nurs Forum. 2001 Apr;28(3):507-12; quiz 513-4. Review. *Erratum in: Oncol Nurs Forum* 2001;28(5):794.

McNeil C. Herceptin in the adjuvant setting: phase III trials begin. *J Natl Cancer Inst.* 2000;92(9):683-4.

McNeil C. Herceptin raises its sights beyond advanced breast cancer. *J Natl Cancer Inst.* 1998;90(12):882-3.

McNeil C. How should HER2 status be determined? *J Natl Cancer Inst.* 1999;91(2):111.

Mendelsohn J. Use of an antibody to target geldanamycin. *J Natl Cancer Inst.* 2000;92(19):1549-51.

Merimsky O, Inbar MJ. Herceptin-taxol related hand and foot syndrome. *Isr Med Assoc J.* 2000; 2(10):786.

Miller JL. Progress in breast cancer treatment: prevention, new therapies come to forefront. *Am J Health Syst Pharm.* 1998;55(22):2326, 2328, 2330.

Miller KD, Sisk J, Ansari R, Gize G, Nattam S, Pennington K, Monaco F, Sledge GW Jr. Gemcitabine, paclitaxel, and trastuzumab in metastatic breast cancer. *Oncology* (Williston Park). 2001;15(2 Suppl 3):38-40.

Miller M. Targeted cancer therapies attempt to hit the bull's-eye. *J Natl Cancer Inst.* 2000;92(23):1878-9.

Montemurro F, Choa G, Faggiuolo R, Sperti E, Capaldi A, Donadio M, Minischetti M, Salomone A, Vietti-Ramus G, Alabiso O, Aglietta M. Safety and activity of docetaxel and trastuzumab in HER2 overexpressing metastatic breast cancer: a pilot phase II study. *Am J Clin Oncol.* 2003;26(1):95-7.

Mordenti J, Cuthbertson RA, Ferrara N, Thomsen K, Berleau L, Licko V, Allen PC, Valverde CR, Meng YG, Fei DT, Fourre KM, Ryan AM. Comparisons of the intraocular tissue distribution, pharmacokinetics, and safety of 125I-labeled full-length and Fab antibodies in rhesus monkeys following intravitreal administration. *Toxicol Pathol.* 1999;27(5):536-44.

Munster PN. Improving breast cancer care. *Cancer Control.* 2002;9(6):455-6.

Murray JL. Monoclonal antibody treatment of solid tumors: a coming of age. *Semin Oncol.* 2000;27(6 Suppl 11):64-70;

Nabholtz JM, Slamon D. New adjuvant strategies for breast cancer: meeting the challenge of integrating chemotherapy and trastuzumab (Herceptin). *Semin Oncol.* 2001;28(1 Suppl 3):1-12.

Nabholtz JM, Tonkin K, Smylie M, Au HJ, Lindsay MA, Mackey J. Chemotherapy of breast cancer: are the taxanes going to change the natural history of breast cancer? *Expert Opin Pharmacother.* 2000;1(2):187-206.

Nagourney RA. Gemcitabine plus cisplatin in breast cancer. *Oncology* (Williston Park). 2001; 15(2 Suppl 3):28-33.

Nagy P, Jenei A, Damjanovich S, Jovin TM, Szölôsi J. Complexity of signal transduction mediated by ErbB2: clues to the potential of receptor-targeted cancer therapy. *Pathol Oncol Res.* 1999;5(4):255-71.

Nagykálnai T. [Evolution of adjuvant chemotherapy of breast cancer from Bonadonna to the taxanes]. *Magy Onkol.* 2002;46(4):307-13. Epub 2003 Feb 1. Review. Hungarian.

Nass SJ, Hahm HA, Davidson NE. Breast cancer biology blossoms in the clinic. *Nat Med.* 1998; 4(7):761-2.

Nelson NJ. Can HER2 status predict response to cancer therapy? *J Natl Cancer Inst.* 2000;92(5):366-7.

Nelson NJ. Experts debate value of HER2 testing methods. *J Natl Cancer Inst.* 2000;92(4):292-4.

Neve RM, Nielsen UB, Kirpotin DB, Poul MA, Marks JD, Benz CC. Biological effects of anti-ErbB2 single chain antibodies selected for internalizing function. *Biochem Biophys Res Commun.* 2001;280(1):274-9.

Nicholson BP. Ongoing and planned trials of hormonal therapy and trastuzumab. *Semin Oncol.* 2000;27(6 Suppl 11):33-7;

Nissenblatt MJ, Karp GI. Bleeding risk with trastuzumab (Herceptin) treatment. *JAMA.* 1999; 282(24):2299-301.

Noonberg SB, Benz CC. Tyrosine kinase inhibitors targeted to the epidermal growth factor receptor subfamily: role as anticancer agents. *Drugs.* 2000;59(4):753-67.

Norton L. Kinetic concepts in the systemic drug therapy of breast cancer. *Semin Oncol.* 1999; 26(1 Suppl 2):11-20.

O'Leary TJ. Standardization in immunohistochemistry. *Appl Immunohistochem Mol Morphol.* 2001;9(1):3-8.

O'Malley FP, Parkes R, Latta E, Tjan S, Zadro T, Mueller R, Arneson N, Blackstein M, Andrulis I. Comparison of HER2/neu status assessed by quantitative polymerase chain reaction and immunohistochemistry. *Am J Clin Pathol.* 2001;115(4):504-11.

Osoba D, Burchmore M. Health-related quality of life in women with metastatic breast cancer treated with trastuzumab (Herceptin). *Semin Oncol.* 1999;26(4 Suppl 12):84-8.

Park BW, Zhang HT, Wu C, Berezov A, Zhang X, Dua R, Wang Q, Kao G, O'Rourke DM, Greene MI, Murali R. Rationally designed anti-HER2/neu peptide mimetic disables P185HER2/neu tyrosine kinases in vitro and in vivo. *Nat Biotechnol.* 2000;18(2):194-8.

Payne RC, Allard JW, Anderson-Mauser L, Humphreys JD, Tenney DY, Morris DL. Automated assay for HER-2/neu in serum. *Clin Chem.* 2000;46(2):175-82.

Pegram M, Hsu S, Lewis G, Pietras R, Beryt M, Sliwkowski M, Coombs D, Baly D, Kabbinavar F, Slamon D. Inhibitory effects of combinations of HER-2/neu antibody and chemotherapeutic agents used for treatment of human breast cancers. *Oncogene.* 1999;18(13):2241-51.

Pegram M, Slamon D. Biological rationale for HER2/neu (c-erbB2) as a target for monoclonal antibody therapy. *Semin Oncol.* 2000;27(5 Suppl 9):13-9.

Pegram MD, Konecny G, Slamon DJ. The molecular and cellular biology of HER2/neu gene amplification/overexpression and the clinical development of herceptin (trastuzumab) therapy for breast cancer. *Cancer Treat Res.* 2000;103:57-75.

Pegram MD, Lipton A, Hayes DF, Weber BL, Baselga JM, Tripathy D, Baly D, Baughman SA, Twaddell T, Glaspy JA, Slamon DJ. Phase II study of receptor-enhanced chemosensitivity using recombinant humanized anti-p185HER2/neu monoclonal antibody plus cisplatin in patients with HER2/neu-overexpressing metastatic breast cancer refractory to chemotherapy treatment. *J Clin Oncol.* 1998;16(8):2659-71.

Pegram MD, Lopez A, Konecny G, Slamon DJ. Trastuzumab and chemotherapeutics: drug interactions and synergies. *Semin Oncol.* 2000;27(6 Suppl 11):21-5;

Pegram MD, Pauletti G, Slamon DJ. HER-2/neu as a predictive marker of response to breast cancer therapy. *Breast Cancer Res Treat.* 1998;52(1-3):65-77.

Pegram MD, Slamon DJ. Combination therapy with trastuzumab (Herceptin) and cisplatin for chemoresistant metastatic breast cancer: evidence for receptor-enhanced chemosensitivity. *Semin Oncol.* 1999;26(4 Suppl 12):89-95.

Pegram MD. Docetaxel and herceptin: foundation for future strategies. *Oncologist.* 2001;6 Suppl 3:22-5.

Penault-Llorca F, Jacquemier J, Le Doussal V, Voigt JJ. [Quality challenge for immunohistochemistry: example of the ERBB-2 status in breast cancer. Group for Evaluation of Prognostic Factors in Immunohistochemistry in Breast Cancer (GEFPICS)]. *Ann Pathol.* 1999;19(4):280-2.

Perez EA, Hortobagyi GN. Ongoing and planned adjuvant trials with trastuzumab. *Semin Oncol.* 2000;27(6 Suppl 11):26-32;

Perez EA. Current management of metastatic breast cancer. *Semin Oncol.* 1999;26(4 Suppl 12):1-10.

Perez EA. HER-2 as a Prognostic, Predictive, and Therapeutic Target in Breast Cancer. *Cancer Control.* 1999;6(3):233-240.

Perez EA. Paclitaxel in Breast Cancer. *Oncologist.* 1998;3(6):373-389.

Persons DL, Bui MM, Lowery MC, Mark HF, Yung JF, Birkmeier JM, Wong EY, Yang SJ, Masood S. Fluorescence in situ hybridization (FISH) for detection of HER-2/neu amplification in breast cancer: a multicenter portability study. *Ann Clin Lab Sci.* 2000;30(1):41-8.

Pestalozzi BC, Brignoli S. Trastuzumab in CSF. *J Clin Oncol.* 2000 Jun;18(11):2349-51.

Peyrot J. Herceptin. *Oncol Nurs Forum.* 1999 Apr;26(3):515-6.

Piccart M. Closing remarks and treatment guidelines. *Eur J Cancer.* 2001;37 Suppl 1:30-33.

Piccart MJ, Awada A. State-of-the-art chemotherapy for advanced breast cancer. *Semin Oncol.* 2000;27(5 Suppl 9):3-12.

Pittsley K. Trastuzumab. *Clin J Oncol Nurs.* 2000;4(5):235-6.

Porterfield LM. Did a monoclonal antibody cause this patient's death? *RN.* 2000;63(9):119.

Pusztai L, Esteva FJ, Cristofanilli M, Hung MC, Hortobagyi GN. Chemo-signal therapy, an emerging new approach to modify drug resistance in breast cancer. *Cancer Treat Rev.* 1999; 25(5):271-7.

Ravdin P. The use of HER2 testing in the management of breast cancer. *Semin Oncol.* 2000; 27(5 Suppl 9):33-42.

Ravdin PM. Should HER2 status be routinely measured for all breast cancer patients? *Semin Oncol.* 1999;26(4 Suppl 12):117-23.

Raymond E, Faivre S, Armand JP. Epidermal growth factor receptor tyrosine kinase as a target for anticancer therapy. *Drugs.* 2000;1:15-23;

Robertson D. Genentech's anticancer Mab expected by November. *Nat Biotechnol.* 1998; 16(7):615.

Roche PC, Ingle JN. Increased HER2 with U.S. Food and Drug Administration-approved antibody. *J Clin Oncol.* 1999 17(1):434.

Saijo N, Tamura T, Nishio K. Problems in the development of target-based drugs. *Cancer Chemother Pharmacol.* 2000;46 Suppl:S43-5.

Sakamoto G, Mitsuyama S. New molecule-targeting therapy with herceptin (trastuzumab), an anti-HER2 (c-erB-2) monoclonal antibody. *Breast Cancer.* 2000;7(4):350-7. No abstract available.

Schaller G, Bangemann N, Becker C, Bühler H, Opri F, Weitzel HK. Therapy of metastatic breast cancer with humanized antibodies against the HER2 receptor protein. *J Cancer Res Clin Oncol.* 1999 Aug-Sep;125(8-9):520-4.

Scher HI. HER2 in prostate cancer--a viable target or innocent bystander? *J Natl Cancer Inst.* 2000 Dec 6;92(23):1866-8. Review. No abstract available.

Scheurle D, Jahanzeb M, Aronsohn RS, Watzek L, Narayanan R. HER-2/neu expression in archival non-small cell lung carcinomas using FDA-approved Hercep test. *Anticancer Res.* 2000 May-Jun;20(3B):2091-6.

Schmid P, Possinger K. [New therapeutic approaches in advanced breast carcinoma. Palliative measures are increasingly more tolerable]. *MMW Fortschr Med.* 2000;142(35):22-4.

Schwartz MK, Smith C, Schwartz DC, Dnistrian A, Neiman I. Monitoring therapy by serum HER-2/neu. *Int J Biol Markers.* 2000;15(4):324-9.

Seidman AD, Fornier MN, Esteva FJ, Tan L, Kaptain S, Bach A, Panageas KS, Arroyo C, Valero V, Currie V, Gilewski T, Theodoulou M, Moynahan ME, Moasser M, Sklarin N, Dickler M, D'Andrea G, Cristofanilli M, Rivera E, Hortobagyi GN, Norton L, Hudis CA. Weekly trastuzumab and paclitaxel therapy for metastatic breast cancer with analysis of efficacy by HER2 immunophenotype and gene amplification. *J Clin Oncol.* 2001;19(10):2587-95.

Shak S. Overview of the trastuzumab (Herceptin) anti-HER2 monoclonal antibody clinical program in HER2-overexpressing metastatic breast cancer. Herceptin Multinational Investigator Study Group. *Semin Oncol.* 1999;26(4 Suppl 12):71-7.

Sibbald B. Making a case for a $2700-a-month drug. *CMAJ.* 1999;161(9):1173.

Slamon D, Pegram M. Rationale for trastuzumab (Herceptin) in adjuvant breast cancer trials. *Semin Oncol.* 2001;28(1 Suppl 3):13-9.

Slamon DJ, Leyland-Jones B, Shak S, Fuchs H, Paton V, Bajamonde A, Fleming T, Eiermann W, Wolter J, Pegram M, Baselga J, Norton L. Use of chemotherapy plus a monoclonal antibody against HER2 for metastatic breast cancer that overexpresses HER2. *N Engl J Med.* 2001;344(11):783-92.

Sliwkowski MX, Lofgren JA, Lewis GD, Hotaling TE, Fendly BM, Fox JA. Nonclinical studies addressing the mechanism of action of trastuzumab (Herceptin). *Semin Oncol.* 1999;26(4 Suppl 12):60-70.

Sparano JA. Cardiac toxicity of trastuzumab (Herceptin): implications for the design of adjuvant trials. *Semin Oncol.* 2001; 28(1 Suppl 3):20-7.

Sporn JR, Bilgrami SA. Weekly paclitaxel plus Herceptin in metastatic breast cancer patients who relapse after stem-cell transplant. *Ann Oncol.* 1999;10(10):1259-60.

Sridhar MS, Laibson PR, Rapuano CJ, Cohen EJ. Infectious crystalline keratopathy in an immunosuppressed patient. *CLAO J.* 2001;27(2):108-10.

Stebbing J, Copson E, O'Reilly S. Herceptin (trastuzamab) in advanced breast cancer. *Cancer Treat Rev.* 2000;26(4):287-90.

Stephenson J. Researchers buoyed by promise of targeted leukemia therapy. *JAMA.* 2000;283(3):317, 321.

Stern DF. Tyrosine kinase signalling in breast cancer: ErbB family receptor tyrosine kinases. *Breast Cancer Res.* 2000;2(3):176-83.

Stockmeyer B, Elsässer D, Dechant M, Repp R, Gramatzki M, Glennie MJ, van de Winkel JG, Valerius T. Mechanisms of G-CSF- or GM-CSF-stimulated tumor cell killing by Fc receptor-directed bispecific antibodies. *J Immunol Methods.* 2001;248(1-2):103-11.

Talukder AH, Jorgensen HF, Mandal M, Mishra SK, Vadlamudi RK, Clark BF, Mendelsohn J, Kumar R. Regulation of elongation factor-1alpha expression by growth factors and anti-receptor blocking antibodies. *J Biol Chem.* 2001 Feb 23;276(8):5636-42. Epub 2000 Dec 4.

Tanner M, Gancberg D, Di Leo A, Larsimont D, Rouas G, Piccart MJ, Isola J. Chromogenic in situ hybridization: a practical alternative for fluorescence in situ hybridization to detect HER-2/neu oncogene amplification in archival breast cancer samples. *Am J Pathol.* 2000; 157(5):1467-72.

Titus K. Another ingredient added to HER2 mix. *CAP Today.* 1999 Nov;13(11):1, 20-4, 26 passim. No abstract available.

Tokuda Y, Ohta M, Suzuki Y, Kubota M, Tajima T. Clinical development of trastuzumab in breast cancer. *Breast Cancer.* 2001;8(2):93-7..

Tokuda Y, Watanabe T, Omuro Y, Ando M, Katsumata N, Okumura A, Ohta M, Fujii H, Sasaki Y, Niwa T, Tajima T. Dose escalation and pharmacokinetic study of a humanized anti-HER2 monoclonal antibody in patients with HER2/neu-overexpressing metastatic breast cancer. *Br J Cancer.* 1999;81(8):1419-25.

Treish I, Schwartz R, Lindley C. Pharmacology and therapeutic use of trastuzumab in breast cancer. *Am J Health Syst Pharm.* 2000;57(22):2063-76; quiz 2077-9.

Tsongalis GJ, Cartun RW, Ricci A Jr. Gene amplification as means for determining therapeutic strategies in human cancers. *Clin Chem Lab Med.* 2000;38(9):837-9.

Tsuda H H. Prognostic and predictive value of c-erbB-2 (HER-2/neu) gene amplification in human breast cancer. *Breast Cancer.* 2001;8(1):38-44..

Tubbs RR, Pettay JD, Roche PC, Stoler MH, Jenkins RB, Grogan TM. Discrepancies in clinical laboratory testing of eligibility for trastuzumab therapy: apparent immunohistochemical false-positives do not get the message. *J Clin Oncol.* 2001;19(10):2714-21.

Valgus JM. Drug update: emerging therapies for breast cancer. *Cancer Pract.* 1999;7(2):100-3.

van de Vijver MJ. Assessment of the need and appropriate method for testing for the human epidermal growth factor receptor-2 (HER2). *Eur J Cancer. 2001*;37 Suppl 1:S11-7.

Vogel C, Cobleigh MA, Tripathy D, Gutheil JC, Harris LN, Fehrenbacher L, Slamon DJ, Murphy M, Novotny WF, Burchmore M, Shak S, Stewart SJ. First-line, single-agent Herceptin(R) (trastuzumab) in metastatic breast cancer. a preliminary report. *Eur J Cancer.* 2001;37 Suppl 1:25-29.

Vogel CL, Nabholtz JM. Monotherapy of metastatic breast cancer: a review of newer agents. *Oncologist.* 1999;4(1):17-33.

Watanabe T, Shimizu C, Katsumata N, Saijo N. [Trastuzumab for treatment of advanced breast cancers]. *Nihon Rinsho.* 2000;58 Suppl:340-4.

Weiner LM. An overview of monoclonal antibody therapy of cancer. *Semin Oncol.* 1999; 26(4 Suppl 12):41-50.

Weiner LM. Monoclonal antibody therapy of cancer. *Semin Oncol.* 1999;26(5 Suppl 14):43-51.

White CA, Weaver RL, Grillo-López AJ. Antibody-targeted immunotherapy for treatment of malignancy. Annu Rev Med. 2001;52:125-45. Review. *Erratum in: Annu Rev Med* 2002;53:xi.

Wisecarver JL. HER-2/neu testing comes of age. *Am J Clin Pathol.* 1999;111(3):299-301.

Wolff AC. Systemic therapy. *Curr Opin Oncol.* 2000;12(6):532-40.

Wong WM. Drug update: trastuzumab: anti-HER2 antibody for treatment of metastatic breast cancer. *Cancer Pract.* 1999;7(1):48-50.

Workman JL. Gene regulation and cancer. Gene regulation and cancer: 10th anniversary meeting of the American Association of Cancer Research Special Conferences in Cancer Research, the Homestead, Hot Springs, Virginia, USA, 14-18 October 1998. *Trends Genet.* 1999;15(1):9-10.

Workman P. Weekly paclitaxel: an effective and well-tolerated treatment in patients with advanced breast cancer. *Expert Rev Anticancer Ther.* 2002;2(6):611-4.

Wu K, Wang C, D'Amico M, Lee RJ, Albanese C, Pestell RG, Mani S. Flavopiridol and trastuzumab synergistically inhibit proliferation of breast cancer cells: association with selective cooperative inhibition of cyclin D1-dependent kinase and Akt signaling pathways. *Mol Cancer Ther.* 2002;1(9):695-706.

Yamauchi H, Stearns V, Hayes DF. When is a tumor marker ready for prime time? A case study of c-erbB-2 as a predictive factor in breast cancer. *J Clin Oncol.* 2001;19(8):2334-56.

Yarden Y, Sliwkowski MX. Untangling the ErbB signalling network. *Nat Rev Mol Cell Biol.* 2001;2(2):127-37.

Ye D, Mendelsohn J, Fan Z. Androgen and epidermal growth factor down-regulate cyclin-dependent kinase inhibitor p27Kip1 and costimulate proliferation of MDA PCa 2a and MDA PCa 2b prostate cancer cells. *Clin Cancer Res.* 1999;5(8):2171-7.

Yu D, Hung MC. Role of erbB2 in breast cancer chemosensitivity. *Bioessays.* 2000; 22(7):673-80.

Zafonte BT, Hulit J, Amanatullah DF, Albanese C, Wang C, Rosen E, Reutens A, Sparano JA, Lisanti MP, Pestell RG. Cell-cycle dysregulation in breast cancer: breast cancer therapies targeting the cell cycle. *Front Biosci.* 2000;5:D938-61.

Zhang H, Wang Q, Montone KT, Peavey JE, Drebin JA, Greene MI, Murali R. Shared antigenic epitopes and pathobiological functions of anti-p185(her2/neu) monoclonal antibodies. *Exp Mol Pathol.* 1999;67(1):15-25.

Zhu XF, Liu ZC, Zeng YX. [*Tyrosine kinase receptor-mediated signal transduction and cancer treatment*]. Yao Xue Xue Bao. 2002; 37(3):229-34.

ABOUT THE AUTHORS

Dorota Bartusik-Aebisher
Professor, Medical Faculty, University of Rzeszów, Rzeszów, Poland
Email Address: dbartusik-aebisher@ur.edu.pl.

Professor Dorota Bartusik-Aebisher is working at The University of Rzeszow in Poland. Professor Dorota Bartusik-Aebisher research is focused on applications of MRI to cancer treatments. Her research interests are the applications of 19F MR to drug tracking and visualization of cancer tissue. She published more than 300 scientific papers and books chapters in MRI field.

David Aebisher
Professor, Medical Faculty, University of Rzeszów, Rzeszów, Poland

Professor David Aebisher is working at The University of Rzeszow in Poland. Professor David Aebisher research is focused on advancement of photodynamic therapy for clinical medicine including the development of devices for localized release of 1O2 to cancerous tissue, and overcoming the limited tissue depth to which current photodynamic therapy can be applied. He published more than 300 scientific papers and books chapters in PDT field.

INDEX

A

acid, 17, 114, 122
acute myelogenous leukemia, 113
acute myeloid leukemia, 16
adenocarcinoma, 10, 21, 32, 34, 35, 64, 79, 94, 121
adverse effects, 46, 68
adverse event, 7, 46
aesthetic, 102
aggressiveness, 1, 3, 15, 107
alanine, 58, 92
albumin, 41
algorithm, 11
alkaloids, 104
alopecia, 72, 110
anaphylaxis, 46
androgen, 62, 95, 115
angiogenesis, 4, 49, 57, 66, 86
angiogenic process, 4
anti-angiogenic agents, 11
antibiotic, 51
antibody, 2, 4, 12, 13, 14, 19, 20, 22, 23, 25, 38, 39, 46, 59, 63, 97, 103, 115, 116, 117, 118, 119, 120, 121, 122, 124, 126, 128, 131, 132
anti-cancer, 67, 103
anticancer activity, 53, 71
anticancer drug, 6, 17, 50, 63
antigen, 46, 111
antineoplastic agents, viii, 47, 101
antisense, 73
antitumor, 10, 28, 47, 56, 71, 83, 103, 116
apoptosis, 9, 53, 62, 79
arabinoside, 52
arrest, 38
assessment, 69
asymptomatic, 46
autoimmune disease, 54
awareness, 105

B

benefits, 4, 67, 103
biological behavior, 47
biological markers, 46
biomarkers, 32
biopsy, 90, 102
blood, 11
blood supply, 11
brain, 43, 60, 83, 100
breast cancer, vii, viii, 1, 2, 3, 6, 12, 13, 14, 15, 16, 17, 18, 19, 20, 21, 22, 23, 25, 26, 31, 32, 33, 34, 35, 36, 37, 38, 39, 40, 41,

42, 45, 46, 48, 56, 57, 58, 59, 60, 61, 62, 63, 76, 77, 78, 79, 80, 81, 82, 83, 84, 85, 86, 87, 88, 89, 90, 91, 92, 93, 94, 95, 96, 97, 98, 99, 100, 101, 110, 115, 116, 117, 118, 119, 120, 121, 122, 123, 124, 125, 126, 127, 128, 129, 130, 131, 132
breast carcinoma, 18, 21, 28, 34, 40, 43, 59, 60, 64, 76, 77, 80, 81, 86, 92, 96, 100, 107, 117, 121, 129

C

cancer, viii, 1, 2, 3, 12, 13, 15, 16, 17, 18, 20, 25, 26, 37, 38, 40, 41, 45, 46, 56, 58, 61, 79, 84, 87, 88, 89, 94, 101, 118, 120, 121, 122, 123, 124, 125, 131, 132, 133
cancer care, 51
cancer cells, 7, 47, 61, 106
cancer therapy, 7, 20, 54, 58, 68, 89, 112, 123, 125
candidates, 5, 63
carcinogenesis, 68
carcinoma, 10, 33, 37, 64, 84, 88, 95, 110, 116, 117, 121
cardiomyopathy, 7, 51, 95, 118
cardiovascular system, 104
case study, 75, 132
cDNA, 70
cell cycle, 38, 53, 57, 62, 88, 108, 132
cell death, 62
cell invasion, 4
cell invasiveness, 53
cell killing, 130
cell line, 5, 15, 20, 21, 35, 36, 49, 57, 64, 78, 79, 88, 103
cell signaling, 68
cell surface, 19, 62
cervical cancer, 106
cervix, 4
challenges, 11, 35
chemical, vii

chemotherapeutic agent, vii, 5, 63, 78, 106, 126
chemotherapy, vii, viii, 1, 2, 4, 14, 17, 18, 22, 25, 26, 31, 32, 41, 42, 43, 46, 56, 60, 67, 77, 80, 81, 82, 84, 87, 96, 99, 100, 102, 118, 119, 121, 123, 124, 125, 126, 128, 129
cleavage, 53, 74, 90
clinical application, 7, 13, 51, 106
clinical trials, viii, 2, 6, 23, 40, 48, 57, 62, 77, 83, 101, 104, 116, 119
collaboration, 105
colon, 70, 106
colorectal cancer, 19, 75
combination therapy, 10, 20, 39, 122
commercial, 27
community, 52
complexity, 11
complications, 4, 54, 104
composition, viii, 1
compounds, 2, 11, 28, 39, 51, 72, 111
conference, 76
congestive heart failure, 75, 90
controversies, 60, 99
correlation, 6, 34, 37, 58, 64, 91, 122
cost, 27, 55, 76
crystalline, 130
cyclooxygenase, 75, 88
cyclophosphamide, 6, 28, 46, 84, 103, 117
cytogenetics, 27
cytotoxic agents, 6, 78, 107
cytotoxicity, 4, 49, 63, 78, 113, 118

D

data set, 114
deaths, 104
degradation, 50
dendritic cell, 4
deregulation, 53, 69
detection, 23, 45, 65, 109, 127

digestion, 109
dilated cardiomyopathy, 7, 13, 18
dilation, 7
dimerization, 68
disease progression, 5, 26, 46, 102
diseases, 7, 27, 120
distribution, 124
DNA, 49, 57, 65, 88, 103
DNA repair, 49
DNA strand breaks, 49, 57, 88
docetaxel, 3, 14, 22, 26, 52, 62, 84, 89, 92, 102, 121, 124
dosage, 51
dose-response relationship, 8
down-regulation, 73
drug delivery, 12, 31, 55, 71, 76, 115
drug interaction, 127
drug resistance, 128
drug therapy, 53, 125
drug treatment, 4
drugs, vii, 2, 3, 4, 13, 16, 17, 19, 20, 21, 27, 35, 50, 57, 63, 77, 80, 82, 88, 89, 101, 104, 119, 120, 121, 125, 128
dyspnea, 55

E

early breast cancer, 8, 25, 26, 33, 41, 99, 123
economics, 33
elongation, 130
elucidation, 62
endocrine, vii, 1, 3, 18, 21, 49, 113
enzymatic activity, 62
enzyme, 21, 109
epithelial cells, 3, 21, 48
epitopes, 21, 132
esophageal cancer, 20
estrogen, 3, 18, 23, 70
Europe, 52, 57, 86, 87, 92
evidence, 3, 17, 40, 49, 62, 127

evil, 32
excision, vii, 102
exposure, 72

F

families, 106
fever, 46
first generation, 105
flavopiridol, 17, 108
flaws, 48
fluorescence, viii, 2, 11, 18, 21, 27, 33, 45, 58, 62, 78, 81, 88, 91, 130
Food and Drug Administration, 128
formation, 61, 86, 103
fragments, 20
fusion, 91

G

gastrectomy, 94
gastric cancer, viii, 2, 15, 16, 37, 38, 45, 70, 87, 88, 94
gene amplification, 2, 5, 14, 15, 36, 38, 48, 58, 62, 87, 91, 109, 118, 126, 129, 131
gene expression, 36, 54, 91
gene therapy, 33
genes, 39, 48, 104
genetic alteration, 109
genotype, 51
glycine, 58, 92
growth, 2, 3, 15, 17, 18, 22, 24, 27, 35, 36, 37, 38, 39, 41, 46, 55, 58, 61, 76, 79, 80, 81, 84, 87, 88, 89, 90, 106, 116, 117, 121, 122, 125, 128, 130, 131, 132
growth factor, 2, 3, 18, 22, 24, 27, 35, 37, 38, 41, 46, 55, 58, 61, 76, 79, 80, 81, 84, 87, 88, 90, 106, 116, 117, 121, 125, 128, 130, 131, 132
guidelines, 32, 92, 109, 127

H

half-life, 50
heart disease, vii, 104
heart failure, 7, 54, 75, 104, 120
hepatocellular carcinoma, 36
heterogeneity, 16
history, 125
hormone, 42, 66, 110
host, 7
human, 1, 3, 14, 21, 25, 32, 34, 38, 39, 41, 51, 62, 78, 79, 80, 81, 84, 87, 91, 103, 115, 116, 118, 126, 131
hybridization, viii, 27, 45, 65, 109, 130
hypertension, vii, 104
hypothesis, 48, 105
hypothyroidism, vii, 115

I

ideal, 7, 54
identification, 74, 80, 105
image, 121
image analysis, 121
immune system, 7, 68, 110
immunogenicity, 50, 58, 71, 92
immunohistochemistry, viii, 6, 18, 21, 27, 33, 36, 45, 58, 59, 62, 78, 81, 91, 97, 105, 125, 126, 127
immunotherapy, 9, 16, 17, 37, 38, 56, 79, 110, 131
improvements, 54
in situ hybridization, viii, 11, 18, 21, 27, 33, 45, 58, 59, 62, 78, 86, 88, 91, 97, 105, 127, 130
in vitro, 6, 21, 48, 58, 78, 90, 103, 126
in vivo, 6, 12, 21, 50, 58, 70, 90, 103, 118, 126
incidence, 4, 26, 48, 62
independence, 120
individuals, 108
individuation, 88
inducer, 62
induction, 4, 49, 122
inhibition, 9, 22, 28, 33, 38, 40, 62, 86, 103, 117, 132
inhibitor, 22, 35, 38, 58, 64, 86, 89, 90, 108, 132
insulin, 55, 64, 76, 117
integration, 9
interactions, vii, viii, 55, 72, 101, 127
internalization, 57, 71, 85
internalizing, 125
interphase, 27
intervention, 109
intraocular, 124
iron, 31
issues, 5, 51, 107, 121, 122

J

Japan, 59, 97
Jordan, 75, 84

K

kill, 113
kinase activity, 74

L

lead, 8, 30, 110
legislation, 27
leukemia, 54, 63, 130
ligand, 3, 23, 61, 79, 108
light, 67
liposomes, 71
liver, 51, 111
localization, 31, 71
lung cancer, vii, 5, 15, 23, 27, 31, 33, 35, 63, 78, 106, 115, 118

lymph, 94, 102
lymph node, 94, 102
lymphoma, 15, 54, 63

M

mAb, 43, 63
macrophages, 71
magnitude, 51
majority, 54
malignancy, 54, 66, 84, 103, 119, 131
malignant cells, 69
malignant growth, 68
mammography, 101
management, 10, 17, 22, 26, 47, 65, 77, 102, 120, 123, 127, 128
manipulation, 112
marches, 118
mastectomy, 102
matter, iv
median, 47, 102
medical, vii, 52, 102
medication, 54
meningitis, 38, 40
mesothelioma, 36
meta-analysis, 87
metabolites, vii
metastasis, 9, 52, 76, 83, 102
metastatic cancer, 34
metastatic disease, 3, 5, 33, 48, 109
methodology, 113
mice, 7, 107
migration, 3
mimicry, 57, 85
models, vii, 2, 5, 14, 71, 107, 115
moderate activity, 26
modifications, 29
molecular biology, 11, 30, 68
molecules, 2, 7, 34, 47, 61

monoclonal antibody, viii, 1, 9, 24, 28, 34, 38, 45, 56, 58, 62, 80, 89, 90, 91, 102, 119, 120, 122, 126, 128, 129, 130, 131
monomers, 61
monosomy, 19
morbidity, 101
mortality, 70, 101
MRI, 12, 31, 42, 55, 57, 76, 85, 115
mutant, 7
mutation, 4, 18, 96
mutations, 66
myeloid cells, 111
myocardium, 34

N

natural killer cell, 78
neoplasm, 104
networking, 61
neutropenia, 72, 110
next generation, 28
nodes, 102
non-Hodgkin's lymphoma, 84
North America, 57, 86, 87
nucleus, 2

O

opportunities, 33
ovarian cancer, 12, 63, 79, 106, 115, 116
oxide nanoparticles, 31
oxygen, 103

P

paclitaxel, 6, 12, 13, 26, 31, 32, 33, 35, 41, 46, 56, 60, 62, 79, 80, 81, 100, 103, 116, 117, 120, 122, 123, 124, 129, 132
palliative, 2, 9, 74, 102

pancreatic cancer, 15, 23, 64, 91, 103, 117, 120
pathogenesis, 4, 54, 104
pathology, 107
pathophysiology, 111
pathway, 37, 114
pathways, 2, 9, 47, 62, 83, 84, 88, 118, 120
patient care, 64
pharmaceutical, viii, 1
pharmacodynamic properties, viii, 45
pharmacogenetics, 27, 33
pharmacokinetics, viii, 50, 61, 101, 124
pharmacological agents, 26
pilot study, 89, 117
plasminogen, 66, 86
platform, 36
platinum, vii, 28, 102, 118
polymerase, 126
polymerase chain reaction, 126
polymorphisms, 109
polypeptide, 3, 20
population, viii, 5, 61, 105
portability, 127
portraits, 23
positive metastatic breast cancer, viii, 6, 25, 52, 68, 77, 79, 80, 92, 108
pregnancy, 86
prevention, 13, 54, 75, 124
primary tumor, 94, 97
progesterone, 23
prognosis, 1, 4, 23, 27, 47, 63, 92, 107
proliferation, 21, 25, 46, 67, 103, 117, 132
prostate cancer, 58, 62, 77, 88, 92, 94, 95, 103, 115, 128, 132
prostate carcinoma, 10, 17
protection, 58, 92
protein kinase C, 33
proteins, 13, 39
proteolytic enzyme, 70
proto-oncogene, 5, 47, 65, 104
purification, viii, 1, 15

Q

quality, 1, 6, 24, 105, 126, 127
quality of life, 126
quantity, 1

R

race, 66
radiation, vii, 9, 17, 70, 102
radiation therapy, vii, 9, 17, 102
radicals, 103
radiotherapy, 33, 71
rash, 55
reactions, 103, 119
reagents, 69, 114
receptor, 1, 3, 13, 18, 20, 23, 24, 27, 31, 32, 35, 36, 37, 38, 39, 41, 45, 55, 58, 59, 61, 76, 79, 80, 81, 84, 86, 87, 88, 89, 90, 95, 104, 116, 117, 121, 122, 125, 126, 127, 128, 130, 131, 133
recombinant DNA, 120
recommendations, iv, 51, 56, 78
recovery, 82
recurrence, 9, 67, 102
regression, 11
remission, 122
renal cell carcinoma, 57, 86
requirement, 3
researchers, 105
resection, 48
resistance, 11, 19, 30, 33, 36, 38, 49, 55, 60, 76, 83, 84, 85, 86, 88, 100, 106, 118
response, vii, 1, 3, 16, 18, 26, 33, 38, 41, 42, 46, 62, 78, 80, 92, 97, 102, 121, 123, 125, 127
responsiveness, 23, 50, 61, 107
risk, vii, 28, 53, 63, 101, 122, 125
risk factors, 28, 72
risks, 46
rituximab, 111

S

safety, 20, 26, 41, 52, 56, 59, 62, 79, 98, 102, 124
salivary gland, 65, 95
savings, 30
second generation, 105
secrete, 11
secretion, 53, 70
sensitivity, 6, 23, 50, 57, 64, 85, 112
sensitization, 60, 100
sequencing, 36, 47, 113
serum, 6, 126, 129
showing, 6, 107
side effects, 52, 70, 103
signal transduction, 2, 9, 14, 40, 53, 55, 58, 68, 77, 94, 125, 133
signaling pathway, 39, 47, 75, 132
signalling, 80, 81, 112, 130, 132
signals, 2, 58, 65, 92
single chain, 125
solid tumors, 45, 63, 77, 106, 120, 124
spleen, 51, 111
stabilization, 62
standardization, 69, 88, 109
state, 10, 16, 48, 63
stenosis, 14
stimulation, 3
stomach, 32
strategy use, 116
stratification, 48
supervision, vii, 115
surveillance, 119
survival, 3, 4, 26, 33, 46, 64, 92, 102, 118
survival rate, 52
survivors, 75, 90
symptoms, 64, 106
syndrome, 124
synergistic effect, 5, 106
synthesis, 17, 114, 122

T

T lymphocytes, 24
tamoxifen, 11, 37, 54, 66, 107, 118
target, 6, 13, 16, 22, 25, 31, 46, 58, 64, 89, 108, 115, 119, 124, 126, 128
taxane, 8, 26, 35, 103
techniques, 11, 69
technologies, 26, 114
technology, 22, 68
testing, 5, 18, 19, 23, 24, 32, 34, 37, 42, 54, 56, 58, 64, 76, 78, 80, 81, 91, 107, 119, 121, 122, 125, 128, 131
texture, 41
therapeutic agents, 15, 27, 72, 111
therapeutic approaches, 2, 74, 129
therapeutic benefits, 30
therapeutic effect, 1, 68
therapeutic interventions, 71, 105
therapeutic use, 40, 84, 119, 130
therapeutics, vii, 23, 53, 58, 94
therapy, vii, 3, 12, 13, 14, 16, 17, 19, 20, 22, 23, 25, 32, 37, 38, 39, 40, 41, 46, 55, 57, 59, 60, 63, 76, 77, 80, 82, 83, 86, 89, 95, 99, 102, 115, 117, 119, 120, 121, 123, 125, 126, 127, 128, 129, 130, 131
thinning, 7
tissue, vii, 5, 23, 27, 109, 124
toxicity, 3, 25, 49, 60, 68, 99, 104, 119, 129
transcription, 21, 107
transduction, 2, 53
transfection, 50
transformation, 4, 17, 27, 47, 61, 91, 107
transitional cell carcinoma, 38
transmembrane glycoprotein, 4
transplant, 129
transplantation, 112
trastuzmab, 45, 61
trastuzumab, v, vii, viii, 1, 2, 3, 12, 14, 15, 16, 17, 18, 19, 20, 21, 22, 23, 24, 25, 31, 32, 33, 34, 35, 37, 38, 39, 40, 41, 42, 45,

55, 56, 57, 59, 60, 61, 62, 76, 77, 78, 79, 80, 81, 82, 83, 84, 85, 86, 87, 88, 89, 90, 91, 92, 93, 95, 96, 97, 98, 99, 100, 101, 115, 116, 117, 118, 119, 120, 121, 122, 123, 124, 125, 126, 127, 128, 129, 130, 131, 132
trastuzumab therapy, vii, 34, 37, 54, 87, 101, 122, 131
treatment, vii, viii, 1, 2, 3, 12, 13, 15, 16, 19, 23, 25, 31, 33, 34, 35, 36, 39, 42, 45, 56, 57, 59, 63, 77, 80, 83, 88, 89, 90, 91, 92, 95, 96, 97, 98, 100, 102, 116, 117, 118, 119, 120, 121, 122, 123, 124, 125, 126, 127, 131, 132, 133
trial, 7, 12, 14, 18, 19, 32, 35, 40, 49, 80, 93, 116
tumor, viii, 3, 15, 18, 19, 23, 24, 25, 38, 42, 46, 61, 62, 79, 89, 90, 92, 94, 95, 102, 118, 130, 132
tumor cells, 24, 25, 42, 46, 70, 89
tumor growth, 28, 38, 71, 110
tumor necrosis factor, 79
tumor progression, 62
tumorigenesis, 27, 67, 83, 84
tumors, vii, 2, 3, 12, 27, 32, 36, 45, 64, 91, 102
tumour growth, 11
tumours, 11, 26, 72

tyrosine, 1, 4, 48, 58, 59, 63, 89, 90, 95, 106, 116, 126, 128, 130

U

United States, 52, 66
urokinase, 70, 86
uterus, 4

V

valuation, 18, 59, 116, 121
vascular endothelial growth factor, 52
vascular endothelial growth factor (VEGF), 52
vascularization, 52
vasculature, 11
VEGF expression, 53

W

Western blot, 65
workflow, 43

X

xenografts, 107, 116